The King's Table

A guide for being up to ten times stronger, happier and healthier.

By Daniel W Osborne with Biblical Daniel.
Edited by Nancy G Walker, Osborne,
Cueto

ISBN-13: 978-1478297345

Made in the USA

To Machelle, my patient wife, and all of my supportive family and to God who gives us mental impressions.

Contents

About this book,   VI

Legal Disclaimer,   VIII

Note,   IX

Epigraph,   X

The Eden diet,   XI

1. Daniel's life in faith and how to connect with God....................1
2. Daniel's diet....................11
3. Give up all unclean foods a beverages....................21
4. How to begin a health diet?....................27
5. Meals....................37
6. How to eat considering personal genetics and exercise....................63
7. Understanding an initial health diet........69
8. Losing weight by lifestyle change.........89
9. The three pillars of better health...........99
10. Self awareness....................127
11. What is moderation? What is healthy?....................135
12. How to consider sources of information....................149
13. Activated charcoal capsules...........159
14. Heal thyself, while doing no more harm....................165
15. Preaching on health....................183
16. More on creating a happy lifestyle..187
17. Life span, count those cell divisions....................191
18. Clean up your environment!....................197

19. Competitive mentality verses adaptive mentality..201
20. Solving your illness problem.........207
21. Ten-day challenges......................235
22. Vitamins and minerals.................247
23. List of common deficiencies.........253
24. Water...265
25. Herbals and homeopathic treatments......................................269
26. Why buy organic?.......................275
27. Cooking is a methodology.............279
28. More on oil and fat.......................301
29. Human history of common foods...307
30. Parasites and Worms...................313
31. Elimination diet program...............319
32. Fasting programs.........................323
33. An introduction to food additives and altered foods............................355

Epilog; Living by Biblical Daniel's example..381
References...387

About this book...

This book is about my personal experiences and research into better health. I do not have medical health insurance. Therefore, I use methods of prevention and gentle healing by natural methods. I personally found this to be a great advantage in my life, to prevent illness or treat it early rather than struggling for a cure after extreme sickness. When feeling sick, natural methods can be helpful in many cases. Instead of letting minor health issues grow, I use natural treatments of diet, lifestyle and herbs to arrest or reverse the condition.

Of course, along the way I experimented, and had successes and failures. Sometimes the mistakes I made are due to a health expert who did not know everything, or I misinterpreted their suggestions. One aim of this book is to show my successes and failures in health, lifestyle and diet, to learn from my experiences. I also include my ideas and research in the area of health and positive lifestyle. I have a Godly aim in some of my writings because I feel anyone with a little faith can draw on this. I feel compelled to help people to understand how a relationship with their higher power may help them in life and health.

I want readers to know what kind of book this is before they borrow or purchase. It is not by someone with a PhD or Doctor title or any other official credential.

I try to be healthy and happy; I am always learning, exploring and trying new things. If this describes you as well, we are traveling on the same path.

In everything, I write I strive to be a direct and honest person. I am an expert in better lifestyle for myself because I have lived and studied this for many years and I am more happy and healthy because of it.

The benefits of learning Biblical Daniel's example and reading this book are...

1. Learn how to be up to ten times better in health, having more vigor, endurance, strength and greater mental ability. This is achievable in a natural long lasting way.

2. Learn how to communicate with God, to pray and listen afterward for mental impressions as plans of action to improve oneself.

3. Learn how to make a diet for better health, and lose weight by following a two meals a day diet lifestyle. And learn how to keep weight off for the rest of your life.

4. Learn to cook healthy tasty food by using simple cooking skills and special condiments. Basic cooking is not about a bunch of recipes.

5. Learn how to detect and eliminate foods and beverages that cause adverse reactions.

And much more...

The necessary legal disclaimer

I am not a licensed healthcare professional (Doctor, PhD etc). This book describes my research, experiences and ideas on health as an interested nonprofessional in health. It communicates my ideas about health, which is unique to me and may not apply positively to anyone. This book is not a replacement for expert licensed medical care. This book is for entertainment use because I may have made unintentional mistakes in stating correct information. In addition, I may have made unintentional mistakes regarding my opinions about diet, health, lifestyle, religion and otherwise.

This book cannot diagnose, treat or cure any health condition. You should seek out multiple information resources in health and lifestyle. You should crosscheck any information source (including this one). You should not take action due to this book without consulting with a license medical care professional and doing further research.

Read this book while intending to take full responsibility for your own actions. Understand that if you are able to comprehend this book. Then you are also able to understand that you assume all risk and liability for all actions you take or not take because of reading this book. Read further only if the statements in this disclaimer are acceptable to you.

NOTE

I sincerely encourage anyone who wants better health and lifestyle to think cautiously about any information and do further research. Even an expert can make mistakes in giving advice, and these mistakes can harm people. In addition, another's personal experience may not be useful, because everyone has a different genetic make up and history.

In addition, an earnest person with a *specific* positive experience over a time, with a diet practice, pill or supplement etc, for weeks, months, even years, may not have a specific negative effect that happens to others. This actually happens often enough, happened to me.

A good practice in health is to read broadly from many sources of information, and to be cautious about anything new, especially with strong effect.

There is a war of information control going on in the diet and healthcare industry, alternative verses conventional. The biggest battlegrounds are on the internet, in the universities in science research and even in the government. Many information sources have money interests tied up with them. You can find information going both ways for most diet and treatment options, conventional verses alternative. If possible, you should talk directly to people who have done the exact health care treatment, lifestyle or diet practice that you are interested in trying.

From the Apostle Paul, First Corinthians, Chapter 3.

"I have fed you with milk and not with meat for you are not able to bear it."

This statement means in a spiritual sense, "To feed a person only what they are able to digest".

The Eden diet

If we look at the story of the Garden of Eden, and afterward, in terms of humankind's changing diet and lifestyle. In the garden, Adam and Eve had fresh foods direct from plants, trees and herbs bearing seeds.

The lifestyle during their time in the Garden of Eden was special. They lived in nature, with greenery all around them, in harmony with animals and ate no meat. Adam and Eve had a strong connection to God and were at peace in a pristine garden. They ate clean natural foods and their beverage was pure water.

Humankind over the centuries has moved farther and farther away from the original diet. The pace of change is accelerating in recent times due to food additives, genetic engineering and countless other ways to make foods unnaturally.

Biblical Daniel's example shows a diet and lifestyle somewhat close to the original one. I think he purposely chose his lifestyle to be healthier and closer to God. By adhering to a Garden of Eden kind of diet, you may be up to ten times happier, healthier and stronger.

Chapter One

Daniel's life in faith and how to connect with God

Daniel 1:8

Daniel purposed in his heart that he would not defile himself with the King's meat nor with the wine, which the King drank.

1 In the third year of the reign of ,Jehoiakim king of Judah came Nebuchadnezzar king of Babylon unto Jerusalem, and besieged it.

2 And the Lord gave Jehoiakim king of Judah into his hand, with part of the vessels of the house of God: which he carried into the land of Shinar to the house of his god; and he brought the vessels into the treasure house of his god.

3 And the king spake unto Ashpenaz the master of his eunuchs, that he should bring certain of the children of Israel, and of the king's seed, and of the princes;

4 Children in whom was no blemish, but well favoured, and skilful in all wisdom, and cunning in knowledge, and understanding science, and such as had ability in them to stand in the king's palace, and whom they might teach the learning and the tongue of the Chaldeans.

5 And the king appointed them a daily provision of the king's meat, and of the wine which he drank: so nourishing them three years, that at the end thereof they might stand before the king.

6 Now among these were of the children of Judah, Daniel, Hananiah, Mishael, and Azariah:

7 Unto whom the prince of the eunuchs gave names: for he gave unto Daniel the name of Belteshazzar; and to Hananiah, of Shadrach; and to Mishael, of Meshach; and to Azariah, of Abednego.

8 But Daniel purposed in his heart that he would not defile himself with the portion of the king's meat, nor with the wine which he drank: therefore he requested of the prince of the eunuchs that he might not defile himself.

9 Now God had brought Daniel into favour and tender love with the prince of the eunuchs.

10 And the prince of the eunuchs said unto Daniel, I fear my lord the king, who hath appointed your meat and your drink: for why should he see your faces worse liking than the children which are of your sort? then shall ye make me endanger my head to the king.

11 Then said Daniel to Melzar, whom the prince of the eunuchs had set over Daniel, Hananiah, Mishael, and Azariah,

12 Prove thy servants, I beseech thee, ten days; and let them give us pulse to eat, and water to drink.

13 Then let our countenances be looked upon before thee, and the countenance of the children that eat of the portion of the king's meat: and as thou seest, deal with thy servants.

14 So he consented to them in this matter, and proved them ten days.

15 And at the end of ten days their countenances appeared fairer and fatter in flesh than all the children which did eat the portion of the king's meat.

16 Thus Melzar took away the portion of their meat, and the wine that they should drink; and gave them pulse.

17 As for these four children, God gave them knowledge and skill in all learning and wisdom: and Daniel had understanding in all visions and dreams.

18 Now at the end of the days that the king had said he should bring them in, then the prince of the eunuchs brought them in before Nebuchadnezzar.

19 And the king communed with them; and among them all was found none like Daniel, Hananiah, Mishael, and Azariah: therefore stood they before the king.

20 And in all matters of wisdom and understanding, that the king enquired of them, he found them ten times better than all the magicians and astrologers that were in all his realm.

The Biblical story of Daniel shows a young man's faith tested to the extreme. He was taken from his home and forced to be a eunuch slave to serve a foreign king, few of us will ever face such a trial. To go against a King in those ancient times would be certain death. Still he risked his life to keep his faith and do what he knew to be correct. He maintained his way of diet and faith in the face of great danger. In those days, many people worshiped multiple Gods with idols. Daniel worshiped a single God. Because of his faith and connection to God, Biblical Daniel and his companions experienced blessings of superior health and abilities.

This book is a highlight of my personal experience and research on health, also my wife's knowledge in health as a fifth generation Adventist, a faith that believes in healthy living. With help from God, I created this book for people to try to live a better life. I believe if you want to be healthier and try sincerely, and ask God for help, he will help if you listen and do what he says. I also believe that if you follow good health practices as like Biblical Daniel, you will be up to ten times stronger in all ways when compared to an unhealthy lifestyle.

I realize some people reading this book may have a different viewpoint of God than a Christian viewpoint. I want to remind that there is no set viewpoint about God even among Christians. In addition, there is a conflicting thought inside the hearts of many Christians; it is strict legalism verses non-strict legalism. In legalism to be close to God, is to focus on a particular notion of Biblical law, verses non-strict legalism where you focus on building a relationship with God. I favor building a positive relationship with God rather than focus on legalism. Often religious legalism can cause people to judge others; thereby they act as if they are a miniature God, which is negative. A person does not need to attend church every Sabbath and appear to "walk the walk", and "talk the talk" to others to be close to God.

Most people have a concept of God in some fashion, there is wisdom in the Bible, and this is true no matter your belief system. I feel like the rules and stories in the Bible are there to help people. For example, if you follow the Ten

Commandments, it will help you in life; otherwise, your life will be much harder. The stories in the Bible are a way for you to better yourself, if you read them in this light.

Many non-Christian people have a concept of a higher power. If this is your situation, you can use your own concept of a higher power while reading this text. I think most people can agree that a positive God does not want people to be unhappy and sickly.

In my experience, answers to prayer may not be what you expect, but on reflection are reasonable. I believe sometimes when people pray for guidance, often for an answer they get a mental impression from God that is not what they expect, so they discard it. Consider listening carefully to the answer God actually gives you. I think often when people pray for help, in time God will impress in their mind a solution or give an outside influence to be the path for a solution. However, they may ignore it, because it is not what they expect. People want a solution that is easy, like a magic pill or something just given to them in some fashion, but this rarely happens.

God gave humankind free will in the world, so God may impress a solution into your mind as an answer to prayer, but he will not force it on you. God may work miracles, but more often he will only impress a solution into your mind for a prayed for problem. Then he expects action from you to gain the desired results, no action, no results. God gave you free will, therefore he most likely will not tell you exactly how to run your life, but he does want to help you in the positive life you choose yourself. God does not want to force people, to eat this kind of food or to live this kind of lifestyle, or even do a certain type of work. Therefore, when you pray to God for help he is less likely to give a miracle without your input. More often, he will impress an idea into your mind illuminating a path of positive action.

A common example is a person eating garbage for food and praying for better health. They are hoping for an unlikely good health miracle. However if you pray and listen when impressed by God to do positive lifestyle changes, positive results are likely to happen. It may be something small like taking a supplement for a while, or something big, like a total change in diet, exercise and lifestyle. I cannot say God always will give relief from all suffering, but I do believe he will help as you pray and make an effort.

There may be a reason for a person's adverse situation and we do not understand why in relation with God. In all cases, there is always something positive to give or gain in the world. One can try to be glad in their heart and enjoy what they do have. I feel bad for those with a physical injury with no cure; nevertheless, most people can work toward a better life with God's help.

God gave us all free will to choose our own lifestyle and activities, good or bad. In addition, God gave all other men free will as well, so if you are having trouble with another person, God *may* impress on another person's mind in your behalf if you pray for it, however that person has their own free will to choose. God cannot force a change inside of people's minds and still give them free will. Free will along with people making bad decisions causes most of the difficult situations and events in life.

For example if you pray for a promotion, God *may* impress something positive into the boss's mind for you. Still, the boss has the free will to choose. Countless other examples are possible. I feel like we are in difficult situations in normal life as potential lessons for us to learn something positive. If so how many of us get the lesson the first time around?

Life can be difficult and bad events can happen to good people for no apparent reason. During life's trials, people can show loyalty, fidelity, faith, honesty, bravery, love, kindness and patience. In everyone's life, there are tests of character. An older person can show bravery when they have an untreatable condition. A child with an incurable disease can show impossible courage. People in great need enable others to show corresponding kindness. People may keep faith while feeling crushing disappointment and adversity.

A person can try to learn positive lessons while praying to God for help during hard times. Alternatively, a person in difficulty can endlessly sin and create an even harder life for themselves and others without trying to be better.

What kind of friends you decide to be around will affect your health and lifestyle. We can choose different friends if we need to. More difficult is dealing with situations that you cannot change easily and God seems not to be helping, or helping quickly enough. These instances are times of life's hardest lessons. I feel like in the majority of cases God will help you, if you sincerely pray and listen for his impressions to act on.

Even when making positive lifestyle choices sometimes-bad things happen to good people for no apparent reason. It is my hope that there is a purpose for this, maybe something positive for someone to learn or just a chance to show character. Such events (maybe tests or potential lessons?) are difficult to accept as being allowed by God. However, more often than not, bad events happen because of poor choices made by the people involved.

A true story, from a woman in our extended family, her child was sick with intestinal problems and she was taking him to be treated, but the doctors could not find a cure for over a week. The situation was getting life threatening. However, she prayed and prayed all this time, eventually she was ready to listen to God's answer. After a mental impression, which she attributes to God, she gave her little boy yogurt and he became well. Of course, she did not expect such a simple solution. She wanted a different kind of answer to prayer, but cure required her action and by faith, she finally listened and acted.

When you pray, listen carefully for the exact answer given and the solution will most often require you to do something. Of course, when praying and listening for impressions from God, use a measure of common sense.

How do you know for sure if God answered you with an impression? We may honestly wonder, "Did a notion pop into my mind from within"? This is the method I use to proceed. Does the impressed solution seem reasonable? Can the solution be tested and no harm done? Alternatively, is there danger of harm from testing the impression? If no danger, then it is safe to go forward when you get a mental impression that you feel is from God.

Safe examples are small diet changes, or taking non-harmful supplements, or changing an exercise program in a moderate way. Alternatively, being open to another's reasonable suggestion, like a doctor talking about a procedure. I cannot name all the possible scenarios that may come up. This is where common sense comes into play and if you are confused, pray some more. It may take patience to wait for an answer. The impression will come; a person or book will appear. *Something* will happen, often quickly, but it may take time.

Of course, I can imagine people doing crazy things and claiming impressions from God, and citing this book, *please use common sense!* For questions about impressions, consult with an open-minded medical care professional of faith. This can be critical for impressions that may cause harm. In every case in my life to date, the impressions I receive can be tested with no danger. If there is danger of harm, then it is unlikely to be from God and it is best not to do it.

I think it is important for a person to do their own active part in health and lifestyle. You should seek out information everywhere, in order to have a knowledge base. It will help in your daily life, and for understanding impressions after prayer.

Another true story, an evangelist came to our local church to give a series of lectures. He told a story about his sick little boy of many years ago. The boy had terrible breathing problems and the family prayed and prayed for a miracle. However, years went by, and the miracle did not happen and the boy became sicker and sicker. During this time, the father had several calls to work and live in a different area of the country. However, he was afraid to leave because of the available near by medical care his boy needed.

Eventually, once again, a call came and this time after much prayer, he decided to risk it. He moved to another part of the country to see how it would work out. Almost instantly, his boy was better after being in this new environment.

Something in the location or home of the original residence was making the boy sick. Maybe it was an allergy to something in that area. No one knows why, but in the new environment, the boy grew up healthy.

Chapter Two

Daniel's diet

The king tested Biblical Daniel and found him to be more healthy and wise than all his men who partake of excess meat and wine. Just about everyone in today's world will be more healthy and wise on Biblical Daniels diet. However, most people are used to an unhealthy diet and lifestyle because they grow up this way. Once accustomed to a poor lifestyle our thinking justifies eating unclean foods. Simply, it is what we are used to.

Popular understanding of what is healthy comes from local community and family. Sadly, popular culture is often wrong. For example, some think to eat much meat is to be physically strong. However, if you fill your gut with large amounts of toxic meat, it may slowly rot and release toxins as it traces back and forth in your intestinal tract, causing slight to extreme illness. Meat eating animals have a short intestinal track to process meat quickly.

Here are the possible causes of ill health due to meat. Excess meat means a lot of protein, which may overstrain the kidneys. Meat may have parasites, especially if undercooked. Meat may have toxins inside of it, because the fat in the meat may have toxins. Meat may have hormones and antibiotics. Rotten meat has the bodies and feces of the bacteria inside it; these are toxic even if you kill the bacteria by cooking.

(It is risky but in a survival situation, you may wash the bacteria and feces away in slightly rotten meat. By flushing the meat three to four times with water while cooking, boiling is the best cooking method to use). Processed meat products such as cold cuts or sausage usually have food additives, which can cause adverse reactions for some people. In addition, the additives used in processed meat can build up to cause cancer, such as colon cancer.

It is not wise to eat unclean meat or great amounts of meat when you have better alternatives. Nor great amounts of wine (alcohol), it is wise to ingest meat and wine in small amounts occasionally and from the cleanest sources and preparation. King Nebuchadnezzar and his royal subjects ate a diet rich in unclean meat, wine and fine delicacies. Their glutinous consumption of bad food and drink dulled their minds and bodies.

We do not know everything the king's men ate in those days, but we do know there was a difference in types and amounts of food between Daniel and the king's men. Daniel and his companions ate pulse. This is food made of fruits, nuts, grains, seeds, legumes and vegetables, made in a plain simple way. This means few spices, sugars, and a minimal amount of cooking to keep nutrition.

Some people of faith eat clean meat such as fish, lamb, beef and chicken in small amounts. To eat large amounts of unclean meat with excessive wine is unhealthy. In today's world, we have additional unhealthy foods and processes to be concerned about, such as pesticides, genetic engineering, refined grains, food additives, excess sugars and modified fats.

Biblical Daniel's strict ten-day test diet was of pulse and water with no meat at all, it is a cleansing diet. I am going to describe transition stages toward a healthier diet. This is more realistic for most people, rather than starting out with a strict pulse foods diet. The idea is to work toward better health in small steps while experimenting with how to eat, and exercise.

Why is Daniel's diet so much better than the king's diet? Alcohol, in quantity is a toxin. Dairy products for many people are toxic. Unclean meat, especially in large amounts is toxic. Pastries and cakes are toxic, especially in large amounts. Modern pastries have food additives and are high in sugar. They have processed carbohydrates and fats in combination. These harmful foods slow the mind, body and erode health until chronic sickness.

The combination of altered fats with processed carbohydrates and sugars clogs arteries and hardens the circulatory system. Unclean meat taxes the digestive system and kidneys. Excess saturated fat in the grain-fattened meat leads to obesity and clogs arteries. Wine (alcohol) in excess is a diuretic, and a dehydration agent, which causes people to loose electrolytes, vitamins, and minerals. In the modern world, we also have soda, energy drinks, coffee, tea, and distilled water that are diuretic in excess.

Caffeine is in coffee, regular tea, chocolate, soda, and in some energy boost drinks. Studies show that caffeine may help with some kinds of short-term mental and physical performance. Research also shows it hurts some types of short-term mental performance. Long-term regular caffeine ingestion can lead to addiction and ill health.

My personal experience is that regular ingestion of caffeine in the form of coffee hurt my overall mental performance. Today, I treat coffee and caffeine as a short-term stimulant. For instance, I sometimes use it when I start to get sleepy while driving in order to stay awake. This works with mixed results because too much may give me the shakes. In long-term usage, caffeine tends to spike up the body's metabolism then it crashes afterward, day after day. This metabolism roller coaster erodes health over time.

For good health the main beverage should be clean water, everything else should be restricted. Normally I drink plenty of water, then sometimes a glass of red clover tea or some other herbal tea. Sometimes I have a glass of flash pasteurized apple juice or another juice.

Most mornings I make a drink of a quart of warm water; inside of it is half of a fresh squeezed lemon. This lemon water is a health tonic because it flushes the kidneys, and lemon is a detoxifying fruit. Sometimes I buy or make juice from fruits and vegetables to drink as a meal or as a midday snack. These kinds of drinks will make one strong and healthy in a steady even way, creating a lasting endurance and strength. This is much better long term than a boost from a so-called energy drink loaded with sugar and caffeine. I would not use caffeine with sugar energy drinks. These energy drinks have little nutrition and will spike up the body's metabolism only to crash afterward. With regular use, they will erode health. It is common for kids to get sick while experimenting with energy drinks.

Let us compare the king's diet to Biblical Daniel's diet. Being faithful if Daniel did *ever* eat meat then only clean meats as identified in the bible and likely in small amounts. If he did *ever* drink wine, he likely did so in small amounts. A modern day Daniel may occasionally drink a glass of wine, possibly with the evening meal. Compare him to the king's men drinking a gourd of wine to get drunk, maybe as a replacement for water and eating lots of meat.

The Biblical account said Biblical Daniel did not eat any meat or drank any alcohol; this is his lifestyle. It is best to drink no alcohol and limit meat intake to clean meats in small amounts. I sometimes ingest more meat than I think best due to social situations and slipping up. When this happens, I often notice an ill health effect and get back on track.

Biblical Daniel probably never ate sweets as we know them, and even if he did so, then in small amounts. He ate a diet rich in natural grains, fruits, beans, nuts, vegetables, olives and plenty of clean water. Since he ate healthier, and was spiritually clean, he was above the king's men ten times in all measured ways. He was not a gluttonous eater and must have had a daily routine in order to eat modestly. Think about your eating habits. Do you eat modestly most days?

2-Daniels diet

During Daniel's ten day fast and the three years of study afterward, he and his companions ate clean foods made of Pulse. They were better than the kings' men in all ways, so clearly you do not need meat for superior health. This goes along with modern human experience; an example is the Chinese Shaolin monks. From an early age, they go through an extreme martial arts training program and are strong and healthy, with a diet totally absent of meat. They eat pulse foods, such as vegetables, rice and fruit; they have a diet similar to Biblical Daniel. They also eat their food in a plain simple way, with no spices. Their protein sources are from plant sources, such as beans, nuts and seeds. Their extreme athletic skills and endurance are an example of the health benefits of a simple diet. On the internet look up the Shaolin monks, and see their strength and health, there are many videos. Their diet and physical training easily puts them ten times above anyone with a poor lifestyle. This is without fancy western supplementation products, meat, steroids, or other drugs.

We may wonder is it actually possible to be up ten times stronger in health and strength? The easiest measurable difference in strength is between being extremely unhealthy and being healthy. It is hard to put a number on how healthier you can be with a better lifestyle, but here is my experience. I know of two people that I grew up with who died in their mid forties due to heart attacks. Both were not fat, but still dangerously clogged up in the heart. I am currently forty-six years old (as I am writing this right now) and not superman by any measure.

But, I know I can carry a 30 to 40 pound pack farther than ten miles while hiking hills. I rarely get chest pains these days and I always feel clear in my heart *as long as I eat correctly.*

For the reader, how do you feel right now? Did you get up this morning right away full of energy with a sharp mind? If yes, likely, you are doing well enough in the days and weeks beforehand in diet and lifestyle, if not, then you have room for improvement. A common situation is that people wake up in the morning slightly hung over due to adverse reactions and later on get their day going-day after day. Poor lifestyle and adverse reactions can be shrugged off in youth, but are more problematic as people age

To start a program toward better health, you need to think about what to give up in terms of bad drinks, foods and habits. To replace these with healthy foods, drinks and habits. Day by day, systematically, this is a never-ending process of self-improvement.

When I was growing up, I was always interested in health but the information sources I had did not include any advanced thoughts on diet and lifestyle. The school system did not go beyond the four food groups. My family ate out of a garden as big as an acre, year around. My mother and father home canned vast quantities of healthy food. I had a somewhat healthy diet as we had good food in general and our family was too poor to buy junk food such as soda and candy. We ate meat, bread, and spaghetti, drank cows milk, everything of the normal American diet commonly considered healthy.

However, as I aged into my twenties, I was able to buy my own food; I started to consume soda and candy in excess. My lifestyle became unhealthy, getting away from garden food toward processed foods and restaurant foods.

The 1990s brought waves of genetically modified foods. In the early 2000s my health was going downhill, I was ready for a lifestyle change. I was not religious in my youth, as my father was not very religious, but my mother is Christen. Nevertheless, I take after my father and still do today in many ways. I grew up in a non-religious household, not atheist, but leaning toward agnostic. Agnostic to me means, "I do not know if God exists and if he does exist, what is he exactly?"

Even today, I still have feelings of agnosticism at times, as I wonder, "What is God exactly?" I think most people; even those of faith have these thoughts at times. As most religious people are always asking questions and searching for answers about God. I do not think these kinds of thoughts are non-normal, that God understands our mystery.

Today, surprisingly for me given my past I am taking after my mother in the belief in God. However, to be honest I am a little agnostic in my faith. Therefore, I do not feel I am qualified to tell others what God is exactly. Nevertheless, I have seen good things happen to me in my life and others that I do not believe are just chance events, I give thanks to God for all his help. I ask for God's help and wait. Often I get impressions and lessons rather than direct blessings, but when so the lessons are a path toward blessings. The lessons are by difficult situations in life I wish I could simply make go away by being suddenly wealthy and healthy, or by some other magical event in my behalf.

I think God often gives blessings through lessons where we should act in some fashion. It works like this; we pray about a problem, God may give an impression as a path to a solution. Then if we act on the impression as God directs, then by this effort and with God's help, we receive the blessing. I see this dynamic happen in my life and others as well. This is my personal viewpoint and experience, I write about this to help people interact with God in a better way-that is my desire.

Why does God interact like this with some people? (I cannot say how God interacts with everyone). I sometimes wonder how it would be if I could talk directly to God. For instance I may ask him,"What should I do with my life?" What would God say? He could tell me exactly what to do of course, but then I would lose free will. I then may ask God "What is the future?" Of course, God can see all, but since, I have free will and so do all other people. Then the future may not be set in stone and it depends somewhat on everyone's actions; if so, what could God say?

What about all the horrible things that happen to people, I may ask "Did he allow these, and if so for what purpose?" I imagine the answer could be too painful and difficult for a human mind to grasp. Then I would ask God about heaven, what would he say? He may show it and it is wonderful, so much so that I would be envious of the dead and possibly wish so for myself.

I do wonder how would it be if I could talk face to face to God and wish I could, but would it turn out well? So far, only mental impressions at times are his answers to my questions, maybe to your questions as well? This seems reasonable to me on reflection. Therefore, this is the situation in my life with God about all things including prayers about health and lifestyle.

I personally think no religious faith has a lock on God's heart, all faiths and people can be close to God or far away, it depends on the person, on their heart.

Chapter Three

Give up all unclean foods and beverages.

Some beverages that should be avoided or limited are coffee, soda, caffeinated tea, alcohol, milk, and sweetened fruit juice. Avoid sugar, saccharine, sucrose, corn syrup, aspartame, and fructose. Most adults should avoid milk. Read all labels on processed food products, if you cannot recognize the word for an ingredient often it is bad, but not always. Replace unhealthy drinks with clean water, herbal teas and the best natural fruit or vegetable juices you can find. One can use a juicer to create fresh juice. You can replace common sodas by buying the more healthy versions from a health food store.

Pasteurization of beverages and food products kills pathogens, which is good, from a public health viewpoint, but this also destroys vitamins and enzymes. An increasing process of today is using radiation to kill pathogens in fruit and other products; the long-term result of this is unknown. I would lean on the side of caution for my family if given a choice. In general, it is best to choose the least harmful processed beverage or food you can find. In other words, choose flash pasteurized juice if you have a choice; this is done with UV light which does less harm to enzymes and vitamins. Buy or make safe non-pasteurized beverages with a juicer whenever possible. Daily beverages need to be as healthy as possible. It makes a real difference over time.

Hot beverages to consume are more healthy coffee substitutes, such as Roma, Postum, non-caffeinated tea, which is herbal tea. Cold beverages to drink are 100% pure fruit juices and water. The best water is clean non-chlorinated water, clean spring water, clean well water, or charcoal filtered tap water. It is better for most people to drink filtered water, I use a charcoal filter on my tap water and it removes chlorine and other toxins.

Foods to avoid or limit are unclean meats, deep-fried foods, all types of common processed cakes and cookies, and refined grain or wheat based products. Most people should avoid dairy. Some products have dairy hidden in them. Watch out for unfavorable oils such as hydrogenated oil, canola oil, soy oil, vegetable oil, palm oil and cottonseed oil. All of these may be genetically modified.

Avoid or limit most pre-packaged foods, even the ones promoted as healthy in a health food store. You need to avoid processed sugar and carbohydrate foods. These cause a shock to the body, because it must digest a large amount of fast digesting carbohydrates. This causes high blood sugar spikes and repeated over time can lead to diabetes and other illnesses. Most people eat far too much of this kind of food and it causes diabetes because the body is not designed for it. Sugars and processed carbohydrates are very easily converted to fat in the body. Therefore, eating breads, cakes, sodas, cookies, brownies and so on makes it harder to keep body weight at normal levels.

A list of Biblically unclean meats is in the

Bible; look in Leviticus Chapter 11. Foremost is avoiding pig meat. Do not eat or strongly limit eating catfish, marlin, shark, swordfish, abalone, clam, crab, crayfish, lobster, mussel, prawn, oyster, scallop, and shrimp. The reason to not eat these is they are unclean animals, scavengers or filter feeders. These meats are more likely to have toxins, parasites, and diseases. The Bible gives this list with the intent to protect your health.   Some people of faith believe that in today's world that only eating zero meat is clean because pollution is everywhere including in all of the world's oceans. I personally think some fish and a little of the cleanest animal meats is fine. However, we do know pollution is everywhere, such as mercury in fish. It is an open question of how much toxin is in the food.

Eat the Biblically clean fish, which have fins and scales. The best fish is clean cold-water ocean fish, and avoid fish farm fish. They are often genetically modified and artificially fed. You can eat fruit's and vegetables, whole grain brown rice or jasmine rice, any natural rice is good. I use rice-based pasta's. Good daily staple foods are beans, oats, olives canned in sea salt, all vegetables, fruits, nuts and seeds, try to buy organic. Whole grain products may be eaten, but be careful as many processed grain products are too finely processed.

Processing breaks the grains down and turns them into high glycemic carbohydrate foods. High glycemic means they digest too fast and may create a strain on some digestion organs, primarily on the pancreas by blood sugar spikes. Many people are allergic to wheat and gluten, it is likely many people have a slight reaction to these and do not realize it. If so, this is eroding their health.   Buying organic is important because pesticides, additives and genetic engineering are harmful.

During transition to better health, buy the better kinds of processed foods, such as cookies, cakes, chips and so on at the health food store. In time, days, months, to years, as long as you need, transition toward eating very little processed foods. During a relapse, it is better to eat a more positive alternative and later on getting back on track. If you have a diet breakdown due to stress, choose a healthier alternative to binge on, and afterward get back on track. This is much better than giving up totally during a relapse.

Oil's: I use olive oil, grape seed oil, safflower oil, sesame seed oil and walnut oil. Olive oil and grape seed oil are good for a salad. Walnut oil is good for baking, olive oil; sesame seed oil, walnut oil and safflower oil are good for sautéing.   Sautéing   is   low   to   moderate temperature cooking using a little oil in a frying pan, if the oil is smoking then it is too hot.

Flax seed oil is an oil supplement taken in the morning, about one tablespoon for every 150 lbs of body weight for health and to curb fat cravings. Eating canned olives is a great way to obtain fat, buy olives canned only in sea salt or healthy vinegar. Avoid lard, margarine, any food with hydrogenated oil or canola oil. Lard is made with pig fat, which may be full of toxins. Most people should limit palm oil and coconut oil. A general rule I have is to be careful about any fat or oil that is solid at room temperature, like lard, palm oil and coconut oil. This is my personal opinion; others may disagree about palm and coconut oil. It may depend on genetics and family history if you can safely eat very much of certain oils, such as palm oil or coconut oil. Note: coconut may be helpful for people suffering from Alzheimer's, for further research. "Alzheimer's Disease, What if there is a cure? The Story of Ketones" by Mary T. Newport, M.D.

An interesting episode, my wife had painful eyes and saw the eye doctor. After the examination, he told her if she were eating coconut oil, it might be clogging up the eye ducts. After she stopped eating coconut products, the condition went away.

Many oils are made from genetically modified sources and this trend is likely to increase into the future. Keep on your toes. In recent years, I notice that many processed cakes and cookies do not have hydrogenated oil on the label because consumers are learning to avoid it. Nevertheless, when I eat a lot of processed cakes and cookies I may get chest pains as if I ate a lot of a product with hydrogenated oil. I suspect there is something in the newer products that is bad for me. The point here is to be careful of all processed foods and pay attention to how you feel after eating. If you feel chest congestion or slight pains in your heart and circulatory system avoid the suspected products or risk a heart attack in time.

It seems to me that the most popular cheap oil of today is canola oil. It is in everything, including foods that are in health food stores. It is used in many restaurants that I have been to lately. Canola oil is genetically created, so is suspicious to me. The cheaper oils in processed foods and restaurants are likely to be genetically altered. I suggest letting others be the test subjects for this grand experiment. Do not be sheep; find out what oils are in your foods and then research to check them out. Bad oils can saturate your whole body in a short amount of time.

Chapter Four

How to begin a health diet?

Step one; Understand God wants you to be happy and healthy, not sick and weak. This is one reason Biblical Daniel's story is in the Bible. Draw on whatever you consider your higher power for daily help. If you desire, find a support group that is into healthy lifestyle.

Step two; Mentally set yourself to be ready to meet a challenge to change yourself, such as a ten-day diet trial like Biblical Daniel.

Step three; Identify your unhealthy foods and beverages and find clean replacements. Examples are replacing coffee with herbal tea and replacing unclean meat with very small amounts of clean meat. The idea is replacing unhealthy items with healthy ones, not just removing them.

Step four; Remove all unclean foods from your environment, and replace with healthy foods. Go through your home and remove all unhealthy processed foods, throw them away. Most processed foods are unhealthy, especially those with food additives. It is best not to bring bad foods home to be tempted.

An initial health diet may not be a weight loss diet; it can be a health change diet, a lifestyle change diet, a cleansing diet. The main goal for diet is first changing eating habits in terms of selecting only the healthiest foods. To create an eating pattern that makes it a habit to have scheduled meals and to snack healthier. This is working toward a better lifestyle. Losing weight is not the first concern for health; the first concern should be to have better eating habits.

The strict Biblical Daniel diet means eating only pulse. A less strict version is very small amounts of clean meat and foods that are not pulse. The less strict version is more realistic for most people to achieve. Which path to take is a choice you have to make. Most will choose to eat a little meat and non-Pulse kinds of foods. For many people eating a little meat is easier. If you decide to eat no meat, you should study the subject and learn how to balance out proteins.

Identifying the addictive or craving foods

If you notice, most fast foods make up the four addictive foods. These foods trigger the desire to eat empty nutrition. Do not get me wrong, the addictive foods are actually good for you, if not eaten in excess and are from nutritious sources. Most convenience foods have some kind of combination of the addictive foods. Some popular fast food items combine all the addictive foods together in one food item.

Here are the addictive foods:

1. Fats
2. Carbohydrates
3. Sugars
4. Salt

These are the big four addictive foods; I would

throw in **Chocolate** and **Caffeine** as undesirable and addictive as well.

I think most people have a weakness for one or more of the addictive foods, by having a craving greater than what they need. *What is your favorite addictive food? Do you have more than one?*

If you observe fast food restaurants, you will often see all of the big four in a single meal, even in a single food item, like a salty biscuit with bacon, and sweet syrup. Usually the easy to buy pre package foods are loaded with one or more of the addictive foods.

What beverages are you addicted to that are unclean? Many people are hooked on soda pop, coffee, caffeinated tea, alcohol, and sweetened drinks. I myself was hooked on a particular kind of soda pop and coffee. For better health, the aim is to replace these with something healthier at a pace you can handle. It is mentally more difficult to remove something from the diet without a healthy replacement. If you do not find a replacement, you have a hole in your life and diet.

Examples: replace soda with fruit juice. Replace coffee with herbal tea. Replacement drinks need their labels read to determine if they are good. A better kind of soda is in the health food store made with natural cane sugar. However, restrict even this kind of soda to a rare treat, as it is still high in sugar. By rare, I mean to transition toward one a week or less.

Drinking a lot of soda pop can cause diabetes in time, depending on genetics how quick this happens. Replacing sugar with artificial sweeteners in soda drinking is no solution. These artificial replacements may cause other health problems such as cancer, fibromyalgia, depression, nerve damage, excessive hunger and headaches. There are more natural sugar replacements such as stevia, raw honey, brown sugar and brown rice syrup. Good natural food is tasty enough without additional sweetness, but many people want additional sweetener because of they have adapted to it. I think all sweeteners should be restricted for the healthiest diet.

Identify all addictive foods, such as foods with excessive animal fat or deep-fried (the high heat needed for deep-frying makes the fat unhealthy). Avoid or limit foods sweetened with white sugar, or most other kinds of sweeteners. Avoid or limit the processed high carbohydrate foods, these can be addicting for some. Avoid or limit extremely salty and spicy foods. Salt in a greasy food can be addictive for some people. I personally think natural cane sugar is less harmful than most other common sweeteners. A good sugar is the low processed brown cane sugar-if you must. Alternatively, there is Stevia, a natural plant based sweetener or raw honey.

Replace processed carbohydrates with natural less processed grain cereals. I prefer whole oat and brown rice based products. If you think you have an adverse reaction to dairy, consider replacing dairy milk with rice milk, or non-GMO soymilk, almond milk, or oat milk. Study the milk products you use to replace dairy milk as they also may have undesirable effects, depending on the product and person. Consider limiting milk use or using no milk at all.

Avoid lard, it is made from pig fat and is a saturated fat. When animals take in toxins, their body may store non-eliminated toxins in their body fat. These toxins will be passed into you when you eat their fat.

Allergen Foods

Common allergen foods many people should avoid, or limit are wheat, (gluten), milk products, peanuts, peanut oil, genetically modified crops, such a soy or corn, find organic versions of corn and soy. Replace peanut butter with raw almond or cashew butter. It is known that peanuts may not be good for long-term health with daily usage. Peanuts most often are roasted and may have toxic mold growing on them. Avoid roasted nuts or seeds of any kind, roasting changes the molecular structure of the oil due to the heat. Raw nuts and seeds are better, buy those made in a plain natural way.

People with arthritis may need to avoid the nightshade family. The nightshades are the tomato, eggplant, potato, and pepper. If you have arthritis, you may have a food related arthritis reaction after eating these. If so, the more you eat the greater the pain and stiffness.

Gluten is inside many grains. The main source is wheat; gluten is a sticky kind of protein, which is not water-soluble. Many people are allergic to gluten, either acutely or mildly. It may glue up your digestive system, especially if you are intolerant. I suspect many people have a bad reaction to high gluten containing foods.

(However, some people who think they are gluten intolerant may be having adverse reactions to yeast or additives in bread products.) Many meat substitute products are high in gluten to give a texture of meat. I personally would eat a small amount of clean meat over gluten filled meat substitutes. Concentrated gluten is very hard to digest.

Many people are noticeably allergic to dairy or are lactose intolerant. I suspect even more have a slight allergy to milk and not know it. An allergic reaction is an adverse immune system response to the milk protein. Lactose intolerant means you do not have the enzymes to digest the milk sugar. It is normal for most people to be unable to digest milk sugar when they get older.

The estimation is that 75% of all adults worldwide are unable to digest milk sugar. This can vary to as little 5% for northern Europeans, a birthplace of using cow's milk, to as high as 90% for people of African or Asian descent. If you are of strong European ancestry then dairy may digest fine for you.

Not all dairy products cause a noticeable reaction for sensitive people because the milk sugar and protein is processed. Explore what you can eat by trial and error. For example, I sometimes eat cottage cheese, butter and yogurt, which I consider the healthier dairy products. The two primary causes of intolerance to dairy are the milk sugar lactose and the milk protein casein. Casein is very harmful when eaten in excess and is in many processed products as a food additive. If you have any slight amount of sinus clogging or phlegm, (flem) problems you may want to eliminate dairy for a while and see how you feel.

Some alternatives to dairy milk are soymilk, almond milk, coconut milk and oat milk. However, these milks are also processed and may be treated with radiation. My wife found she has a noticeable adverse reaction to most dairy milk substitutes, except for oat milk and almond milk. These days we drink little of any kind of milk product because all are manmade and processed.

Allergic reactions are immune responses to proteins. If you have an allergic reaction to one type of common allergen, it is likely you will have others. You can gain new noticeable allergies, while aging because most people become more sensitive as they age. It is a difficult problem in health to figure out the causes of multiple allergies and eliminate them.

In addition to allergic reactions there are adverse reactions, these are bad reactions to environmental items, foods or drinks etc, which are not due to proteins. As a practical manner, an adverse reaction *could* be interchangeably called an allergic reaction. Technically, allergic reactions are harmful reactions to proteins, and adverse reactions are other kinds of bad reaction to foods.   In this book, I consider adverse reactions and allergic reactions to be interchangeable, so that both terms will cover both types of bad reaction.   There are many kinds of allergic reactions due to proteins. In addition, there are other adverse reactions not be forgotten simply because they are not due to protein.

To find the cause of an allergic reaction, one way is to eliminate all suspected items for a time and then add them back one at a time to figure out what is going on. This is especially difficult for those items that need several days of build up time to start a noticeable negative affect. Some people are more mind-body aware than others. Such problems are especially difficult to deal with in children.

Children may learn to be "allergic" to items that they do not like, to the chagrin of parents. In addition, children may be able to shake off slight ill feelings to allergen food items. A parent must carefully observe cause and effect due to foods and beverages, and do careful experimentation. The best practice is to have a clean non-processed foods diet, then watching for bad reactions to normally healthy items that a child may eat. In truth, often even health conscious parents may feed kids items they are allergic to the whole time they are growing up. Professional medical help is advisable to search out allergies with no known cause. Look for a professional in ecological (allergy, nutritional, environmental) medicine for *any* unsolvable mystery illness.

Modified organism (GMO) foods are a concern, GMO causes foods to change rapidly and one may gain a new negative reaction to a food due to GMO. Monitor your health, as foods are changing all the time. A food that you ate fine for years may suddenly cause adverse reactions due to GMO changes, food additives, pesticides and other treatments. It is possible to have negative reactions so slight that you can hardly tell them, and they are slowly eroding health.

Sometimes reactions get more acute as you age or as you eat more of the offending item. The digestion system becomes less effective as people age and this makes allergic reactions more noticeable.   In addition, parasites, toxins and diseases build up so that allergic reactions become more severe.

Chapter Five

Meals

Find healthy sources for these craving foods.

1. Salt   2. Sugar   3. Fat   4. Carbohydrates, and also for protein.

Breakfast

Select healthy foods from each group first thing in the morning. The fat craving can be strong during a new health diet because many people try to restrict fat and oil too much. This is because they originally ate fats from unhealthy sources and did not find healthy replacements; this will lead to diet failure. The solution is to replace bad fats with good sources of fat.

If needed, consider buying flaxseed oil and take one tablespoon per 100-150 lbs of body weight first thing in the morning (one tablespoon has 14 grams of fat). Check the health food stores for other fat supplements such as primrose oil, fish oil and others. However, as a practical manner you can get all necessary oil or fat from healthy raw foods and home cooking. Daily-recommended fat intake is around 40 to 100 grams a day, depending on body size and if wanting to lose weight or not.

Raw nuts and seeds are a good source of needed fat. A half a cup of mixed nuts and seeds will provide 40 grams of fat, which is about 1/2 to 7/8 of your daily needs for fat. An avocado will provide twenty to thirty grams of fat, which is about 1/3 to 5/8 of fat needed daily. For additional fat, use healthy oil in salads and cooking. For instance, put one tablespoon of walnut oil in a salad for 14 grams of healthy fat.

When experimenting with oil and fat sources watch how you feel in order to detect adverse reactions. I personally find that sometimes I do not react well to oil that is supposed to be good for me. This may be due to variations in the quality of processed products. I use how I feel as the final guide in determining weather to keep using a product or not.

A refreshing morning drink is one half to one fresh squeezed lemon in a quart of warm water (I do not favor using lemon juice because it is processed). Drink the lemon water and wait around 15 minutes before eating breakfast. This tonic hydrates the body and flushes the kidneys. I do this most every morning and feel the benefit.

Carbohydrates for breakfast are cereals or breads made from oatmeal, brown rice, jasmine rice, barley, millet, buckwheat, and grits. It is best to cook these from scratch and not use processed packaged breakfast cereals of any kind. If you have trouble with gluten, try cooked rice or millet for breakfast, adding in fruit, nuts, and seeds. Gluten free oats may work for you.

Fats for breakfast are flaxseed, primrose, olive, grape seed, safflower. One can use these in foods or as supplements. A little organic butter at times is fine. Stay away from margarines, because most are made with unhealthy fats and all are processed. Vegetable shortening is likely made from coconut or palm oil; I limit its use to coating baking pans.

Good sugars for breakfast are fresh organic fruit, frozen fruit, unsweetened canned fruit, raw honey or dried fruit. For fresh fruit, scrub the outside skin with a kitchen scrubber. Frozen fruit is great for putting in hot cereals to cool them down, or to create a breakfast smoothie. Watch out for food additives on dried fruit that may or may not be on the label. I sometimes get an adverse reaction from certain types of dried fruit, which should not happen.

For concentrated protein eat raw organic nut butters, (I avoid peanut butter) organic brown eggs, brown beans, small amounts of clean fish (non-GMO, no fish farm). Limit eggs to four to seven a week, I know from personal experience that it is easy to eat too many eggs. In my case, I can get heart congestion and higher blood pressure. If you have heart problems and high cholesterol, consider limiting whole eggs to fewer than four a week. Egg yolk is just one source of cholesterol. Saturated fat is also a source of harmful cholesterol. The most dangerous source of harmful fat is from altered oils inside processed foods such as store bought cakes and cookies.

Store bought egg whites are excellent protein and have little cholesterol. Alternatively, you can boil the eggs and discard the yokes, consider this if you have high cholesterol and want more egg based protein. However, a slightly high cholesterol number may not mean a serious health problem as people have differing normal levels of cholesterol. Cholesterol can be the body's response to inflammation due to bad foods. Do not treat a symptom (inflammation) with drugs, herbs, homeopathies and supplements, while forgetting the cause (bad foods). Feel your heart and circulation system. Do they feel clear or clogged?

A self-done stress test is to walk uphill, you may carry a backpack for greater strain, *but use some commonsense.* Get your breathing up a little, do you feel clear in your heart and chest area. Alternatively, does it feel congested and painful? If painful or congested, it is likely you need to clean up your circulatory system by changing diet. After about a month of better diet, do the test again. You should feel better in the heart and chest area. For any question, see a licensed medical care provider.

In my personal experience, you must be very strict in diet to clean up the circulatory system, and that lecithin and hot peppers help. If you will not keep a strict clean diet, it is extra important to take the prescribed drugs for heart problems. It is far better not to wait until after the first heart attack to make diet changes, you may not survive it. After a heart attack, the damage is done and you are unlikely to heal back to full strength. You will be aerobically weaker for the rest of life.

I have good results taking aspirin for short-term instances of chest pain. However, aspirin is not a cure for heart congestion. It is not healthy to take aspirin daily. The real cure is simple, most people are having chest pains due to eating garbage foods, and the cure is to clean up the diet. For me chest pains are usually because of some kind of modified oil or additive inside a processed product. A person may take one or two aspirin to relieve short-term chest pain and congestion. In addition, they can ingest an amount of lecithin (around 2-4 of tablespoons a day) and hot peppers and clean up the diet. If your heart is congestion sensitive, you cannot eat even a little amount the bad foods. *You must eat a zero amount of garbage foods or risk heart attack and other illnesses.*

Some people seem to handle the garbage foods better. It depends on genetics. Others seem to be very sensitive; these people are more likely to die of heart attack in their thirties to forties unless they have a strict health diet. A strict health diet means little eating in restaurants and zero eating of common store bought processed cakes, cookies and candies. It means mostly eating homemade foods from non-processed organic sources.

It is difficult for most people to believe that a sensitive person has to be so strict in diet and lifestyle to keep health. For me, a few of the very bad processed foods eaten in a week will start to cause chest pains. If clean diet is not enough, which it usually should be (if it is truly clean), but if not, a further step up is fasting to clean out the crud.

Lunch

Boxed lunch: When packing a lunch choose foods that are part of the four craving food groups. Use healthy beverages, such as pineapple juice, prune juice, grape juice, tomato juice, rice milk and almond milk. Make a sandwich from rice bread or spelt bread, or any healthy bread with nut butters, healthy jams, sliced avocado, tomatoes, and rice or soy cheeses. Bring along olives, a can of green olives is good.

Bring unsweetened canned or fresh fruit, raw nuts and seeds. I like boiled eggs with sea salt, sliced tomatoes with sea salt, avocados with sea salt, cantaloupe is good with sea salt. Two condiments, veganaise and pimento cheese will help the flavor and health of lunch food.

Veganaise, can be bought or homemade. Pimento cheese has to be homemade to be healthy as of this writing. The recipes are in the cooking section of this book, page 295. You can buy veganaise in many health food stores. I do not buy the kind made with canola oil; choose those made with olive oil or grape seed oil.

Restaurant lunch: When eating out, choose carefully the restaurants and the foods in them. Find restaurants that offer a menu with a choice of healthy items. I look for Asian, Mexican, or buffet types of restaurants. Stay clear of excessive grease, hardened fats and over cooked foods. In the restaurant, stay away from suspect sauces, dips and gravies. In Asian restaurants look for brown rice, low amounts of meat, and lightly cooked vegetables such as steamed vegetables.

A scary trend in recent times is genetically modified cooking oils. They are everywhere. Guess what the cheapest oil is? I personally avoid vegetable oil, hydrogenated oil, soy oil, canola oil, corn oil, cottonseed oil (cottonseed is considered a vegetable and can be in vegetable oil) and palm oil. I noticed many health books do not have the guts to point out genetically modified oils. That is a shame because you can have perfect food ruined by bad oils. Many oils are modified these days; this is extremely dangerous for personal health.

Some of these modified oils may be safe to use long term. However, I feel that only long-term evidence can be trusted, at least many decades of safe usage, so let someone else be the lab rat. When eating in restaurants, the fruits and vegetables can be good, the small portion of meat clean, however toxic oils and condiments may grind down health. Avoid excess cheese and meat, and choose beans that are whole rather than re-fried, which may contain lard or unhealthy oil. Bad greasy foods can clog up the circulatory system and cause heart pain.

When eating out be aware that some buffets use MSG or other preservatives. Choose the healthy items off the buffet, like rice and vegetables and very little meat, I recommend no pork, a Biblically unclean meat. Egg rolls taste great, but are usually deep-fried, it is best to limit them.

When I eat at a restaurant buffet, I try to avoid items that may have been set out for multiple days, like the soups, or any rarely eaten item. I am careful with the oils and sauce blends, I avoid deep fried food. Eating out is sort of like tiptoeing through a minefield. Recently after eating at a restaurant buffet, I got sick that night and the next day, I suspect a single sparerib that I ate. I wonder how many days it sat out!

In recent times, I find that most often restaurant eating has bad results the next day for me. Someday I may have to avoid eating out almost totally.

Lunch at home: this should be easy for you because all the un-clean foods are out of the house, if not start throwing away now! Here are some good examples of a homemade lunch: beans and rice, these should always be on hand because they are staple items. Steamed vegetables, soups and healthy crackers with a non-dairy dip or spread. Be careful of butter and margarine substitutes, read the ingredients checking for bad oils. You are safe to choose raw or frozen fruits and vegetables, raw nuts, seeds and a healthy drink of some kind.

Dinner or Supper

For dinner, staple items will be beans of different varieties, along with brown rice and vegetables. A salad with fresh vegetables and dressing made of olive oil and lemon juice. Fruit of any kind is great for all meals. If you eat meat, select only low fat meat, such as fish, lamb, lean beef, chicken, fish, and turkey. Hormone free, free range lean meat is the best.

Common livestock meats are grain fed with hormones and antibiotics; these fatten animals in an unnatural way. Better is the grass fed livestock without hormones and antibiotics. The natural color of meat when set out in the air is brown, if it is bright red, dye may have been used. Natural meat is leaner and tougher. One can find it in health food stores in the form of hamburger.

A person who wants to be like Biblical Daniel will eat no meat. Alternatively, a person may eat small amounts of clean meat, one to two times a week or less. I have the best overall health when I eat meat rarely, once or twice a month or less. I do find that recovery from hard exercise may be slow at times and I feel like some meat protein is helpful. For me eating meat is a trade off. Getting concentrated protein verses the possible risk of toxins inside of meat. To understand this if you eat vegetarian the feces smell is very slight, when eating excess meat (and other toxic items) this smell will increase due to the rotting meat in the feces. For me it is healthier to have the cleanest meat and eating very small amounts-when I indulge.

I avoid eating the filter feeding sea animals, because they feed by filtering out the water. They are likely to pass toxins on into you. Examples are crabs, shrimp, scallops, clams, oysters and mussels. It also depends on how clean the water is where the animals come from. Remember toxic waste from humankind is passed out into the sea from bays and rivers.

Snack foods.

When the hunger bug strikes are you prepared? Always have something with you to eat, and not be tempted to buy junk food. Keep raw nuts, fruits, vegetables, olives and small cans of fruit juice. Even a glass of warm water will help during a hunger pang. I enjoy drinking a tea made from red clover blossoms. It is something pleasant in-between meals.

Never let yourself get so hungry to eat bad food. If you feel the crushing hunger to reach for anything, it is best to have something good on hand. For example, there are many types of more healthy ice creams, such as the rice and soy alternatives. They are tasty and mostly guilt free. For best health, in time you will limit even these, but in transition, they are fine. The same can be said about any kind of processed treat item. Buy the best form of it you can find, and work on transitioning all of them out of the diet. You can have them for rare treats for the best health.

Natural treats that you can have all the time are fruits and dried fruits. Often snacking is due to cravings for fats or carbohydrates. If this is the case then eat healthy forms of fats and carbohydrates. If you do not replace the bad with something good, your diet program will fail.

There are many types of more healthy cakes, candies and cookies to choose from without missing taste. I suggest going to the local health food store and cruise the isles for tasty snacks. If the urge hits for a big binge due to stress you can sort of stick to a health diet by always having a variety of the more healthy types of cookies, cakes and candies on hand. Better yet, buy them only when the strong desire hits. If you cook, then it is better as you can make healthier snack items. One can make tasty oatmeal cookies with dried fruit and nuts. These are great for snacking during your transition toward best health and are guilt free.

In time, you will be able to reduce even the healthier made processed snacks close to zero-if this is your desire. These days I eat very little ice cream and the healthier store bought cookies, years ago when starting out I ate these often. I will give you a common situation; let us say you are starting out from a poor diet. Most people eat some healthy foods, moderate amounts of meat and too much of the bad processed foods. Many people drink too much coffee, sodas and have other bad health habits, no matter if they know it or not.

Maybe you have not been feeling well in recent years, possibly you are overweight and try to exercise, but it is not going well. You do not feel good. You think about changing your diet and nutrition toward something better. You can do it, think about creating a method of transition. Little steps to where you want to be, to the body and lifestyle you want to have.

Restrict late night snacking. It is best not to eat within four hours before bedtime. If you follow this rule, you will sleep better at night and have a bigger appetite in the morning. The body needs to concentrate on healing and the digestion organs need time to clean out food. It is healthy to be a little hungry at bedtime. I personally notice a positive health improvement when I follow this practice.

During transitioning toward better health, a good evening snack is berries with healthier ice cream. Berries are especially good for you and the ice cream makes it a tasty treat. Most people should avoid dairy ice cream, choosing alternative ice cream.

For best health, do not eat after the evening meal, but on occasion it is fine when you need. If so, it is better to choose something light like fresh fruit as a snack after the evening meal.

Honestly, I still grab a late evening snack on rare occasions. It is not the end of the world, but most of the time I do not, and that slight empty stomach feeling is telling me that my digestion organs are resting. I sometimes drink a large cup of herbal tea in the evenings to fill my belly with a pleasant warm liquid.

Personally, I found that even the more healthy versions of ice cream, cookies and cakes affect me negatively. Most likely, it is because of the processing and food additives etc. It is better for me to make a homemade natural snack. For example, a homemade smoothie is wonderful; just blend frozen fruit and organic bananas. Add in a little fruit juice to get it started in the blender.

The main thought when starting out is not to restrict the amount of food eaten. It is to the change foods and drinks you ingest toward something better, gradually, the best you can. Later on, only when ready start to control eating patterns to eat less overall, if needed. This transition time can take months to years. It is up to the person and their nature. For most people, it will take a year or more to get a health diet program solid, when starting out with an unhealthy eating pattern. Many people will naturally lose weight just by eating healthy pulse foods, even when eating all they want.

Carbohydrates, fats, proteins

Baking vegetables such as squash and sweet potatoes is very nourishing and high in vitamin A. When preparing to bake, apply olive oil and salt. Spaghetti and lasagna made from brown rice pasta are great occasional dinner entrées. I recommend whole wheat processed products or even better are the brown rice processed products. It is best to give up most pre packaged grain products, and cook from scratch from source grains. This means food that comes out of bins or sacks from the natural foods section of a store. Alternatively, select organic foods as close to the original non-processed form as much as possible.

I suspect many people are allergic to gluten, food additives or yeast in regular bread and not know it. I consider sprouted bread flour to be better, or spelt flour bread, or rice flour bread. For my wife and me, we have the best health if we limit all kinds of bread to a few slices a week. It makes a real difference for us. Look for bread made simply and cleanly, local bakeries may be your best chance.

Remember to fill yourself up with good healthy foods from each of the four craving food groups. You will feel satisfied and the cravings for junk food will be less. If a craving does happen, always have healthier alternatives on hand to relieve it.

Think about what you are craving. Do you crave a type of food more than you should? Do you crave carbohydrates or salty foods, maybe you crave fatty foods, or is it sweets? For each person it is different. Maybe you crave differing combinations of the big four; if so, seek out healthier alternatives.

If your body craves something, it can be an allergen food or something your body actually needs. Know the difference. The body can be craving something not good for it. I think chocolate in excess is not good for health. Therefore, I eat chocolate as a rare treat.

An addictive relationship to a food resembles a drug addiction. You crave it and may feel down without it. Then get high when you ingest it and crash a little or a lot sometime afterward. This is the general pattern.

It is common to go on a health diet and then restrict saturated fat, but a little saturated fat in the diet is not harmful. It can come from eggs, clean meat or organic butter. It is important to ingest enough healthy fat in a diet. Healthy unsaturated fats are from plant sources. Examples are green olives in sea salt, avocados, raw nut butters, raw nuts or seeds, flax oil, grape seed oil, olive oil, primrose oil, grape seed oil and sesame seed oil.

Choose sea salt over regular salt because sea salt has minerals, regular salt has little to none. Sea salt is in most food stores. Some brands have added iodine, which is a good option. If you are very active and sweating, you need salt, apply salt into your food while cooking. Sometimes people on a health kick restrict salt too much. This is unhealthy and can lead to a health crisis. Cramping of muscles is an indicator of low salt, (although cramping is often from other causes) also faintness and weakness. On the other hand, too much salt can lead to kidney strain and high blood pressure. About 1/4 teaspoon in food a day per person is about right. Note: a large amount of salt all at once can dangerously shock the system.

People need protein every day because it cannot be stored up, but it does not have to be animal protein. It is good to eat small amounts of protein each mealtime. Beans and rice are a complete protein source. Some active health practitioners use store bought protein mixes. If you do, I recommend using vegan rice protein or any easily assimilated liquid protein. High protein diets over a long period are hard on the kidneys. It is possible to elevate protein intake slightly to recover from a hard workout while drinking plenty of water. Short periods of time eating an elevated amount of proteins are tolerable for most people. For long-term organ health, I consider it better to eat natural vegetable sources of protein. These days I personally would eat more clean meat over using protein mixes.

An athlete in training needs more nutrition, as well as anyone doing hard physical work, but this may accelerate aging. Consider how much food is needed to maintain current exercise levels-verses long-term health goals.

The better choice for long life is to not use protein powders or eat excess meat and other nutrition. It is best to have moderate food intake if you want to live as long as possible in good health. A healthy excessive meat eater, their lifespan may be restricted to the seventies.

Supplements are made by processing and likely to be hard on the organs. I urge strong caution with their usage. They may harm an organ or organ system over a long time and reduce lifespan. Protein supplements may harm kidney health if used for a long time (months to years), especially if used in excess,

A great protein condiment for all home meals is Braggs Aminos. It is healthy, full of protein and tastes like soy sauce, you can find it in health food stores or order it online. Another great natural protein source is Nutritional Yeast; it has all the B vitamins, and tastes great in food. Many stores carry it.

Mixture of Proteins, Fats, Carbohydrates

Consider the proper mixture of protein, fat and carbohydrate at a meal. In the last hundred years, modern humankind has gotten too far from the maker's diet For instance, take today's processed grains and sugars that are abundant and cheap. The design of the human body is not for digesting so much unnatural food and keeping health.

For example, when eating a high carbohydrate meal made of processed grains, this type of grain digests very quickly. The body responds with large amount of insulin and then depending on genetics the body will crash. This roller coaster ride is more intense with large meals high in sugar and processed grains.

To avoid this, we need to stay away from most processed foods and at each meal have a balance of proteins, carbohydrates and fats. The mixing of proteins, carbohydrates, and fats at mealtime sets the body's response to food to be more tempered. Overall energy levels are stronger and stable; it is easier to loose weight and keep it off.

The proper ratio of carbohydrates to protein is about two to one in calories. The ratio of carbohydrates to fat is also about two to one. It is helpful to have all three in meals to keep the system in balance. This calorie balance is about 45% to 65% carbohydrates, 20% to 35% protein, and 10% to 25% fat.

Rather than measuring out grams of protein, I personally find it best to feel my body's need for protein on a daily basis; if I am doing hard workouts, I add extra protein to my diet along with other nutrition. Unless you are an athlete or doing hard physical work, the need for protein is modest.

As a practical manner if you want to be moderate in meat intake, think about using the palm of your hand as a guide. Imagine taking your hand and cutting off the fingers and the thumb, then cut the hand off at the wrist. After this, you have a whole palm of the hand, and then cut this in half. This half palm is your gauge. Do not exceed this size in meat for any given day.

For a visual guide for proportions, you want to eat a large portion of fruits, grains and vegetables (complex carbohydrates), then a smaller portion of protein, about 1/4 in comparison to the complex carbohydrates. Put in about a 1/2 tablespoon to a tablespoon of oil per person per meal.

For carbohydrates, you want low amounts of processed food items because they are quickly assimilated and will put a sudden shock on the system as compared to natural foods. An example is pasta, especially white wheat pasta. It should be avoided, instead use whole wheat or brown rice pasta. Likewise, for breads, use the whole grain or sprouted grain breads. White potatoes are natural, but are almost like processed grains in the carbohydrate shock they give. However, white potatoes are fine in moderation. My wife and I prefer the red-skinned potatoes. Sweet potatoes are healthy, but also mid to high range in glycemic index.

In general, we want natural foods that will digest slowly while avoiding the processed grain/sugar products that digest too quickly. In addition, many people are allergic to processed wheat products because of gluten, or food additives. This indicates many people are not able to handle gluten, the same for milk products. In short be careful of any food product with a relatively short human history of usage (for your genetics), and are made white by removing nutrition and are super easy to digest. Yogurt and cheeses may be tolerable to people who cannot drink milk, but they should be careful of slight bad reactions eroding health.

Meat is about 7 grams per ounce and a person's half palm is about three ounces in size, this is about 21 grams of protein. This is enough meat protein a few times a week, especially when you add in vegetable protein. I am talking about a long-term health diet, rather than a short-term body building strength program. For long-term health, it is best to have limited food intake. Many can live into their 70's, but to make it beyond this age most people need an easy on the organs diet program.

Hard training athletes and heavy workers need more protein than light exercisers. I caution that if you choose to exercise extremely hard, the needed protein and food may shorten lifespan.

Moderate exercise is healthy when you gain full recovery and not need large amounts of food. Understand, even if excess food is clean and healthy, it still takes extra effort for the body to recover, so this may reduce lifespan. Extreme exercise will likely increase the rate of cellular divisions, which means faster aging.

Glycemic Index.

The glycemic index is how your body responds to a certain kind of carbohydrate food. The way this index is created is by setting pure glucose at a value of a hundred, and then in a trial have test subjects eat different foods to measure their insulin secretion. The higher the insulin response, the higher the glycemic rating of the food, with few exceptions the highest ratings are from the most processed foods. Processed foods and sugary foods cause a disastrously high insulin reaction.

Note: people have varied reactions to hi glycemic rated foods. It breaks down like this; about 25% of people react strongly with pancreas-produced insulin to high glycemic foods. About 25% of people have little reaction and 50% of people have a middle range reaction. Most people who have large insulin reaction to high glycemic foods are overweight. The skinny people tend to be in the 25% low reaction group. The mid range people tend be in the middle of the road between these extremes with variations of weight due to diet and exercise.

Most people tend to be healthier if they avoid large amounts of the high glycemic foods. These are mostly processed foods. If you want to keep weight off, eat pulse foods and avoid products made of processed grains and sugars.

For diet, it is hard to give a blanket recommendation on how to eat. It depends somewhat on genetics. About 25% of people tend to handle high glycemic foods fine and do not get the high insulin spike. These people tend to be thinner. Instead, let us concentrate on the 25% of people who have the biggest problem with these foods and tend to be overweight.

In ancient human history, people had times of feast and famine. During a feast, a high insulin reaction to glycemic foods would enable these 25% overweight people to put on body fat, for a later famine. Insulin causes the body to put on fat for lean times, a great trait in those past days for this 25% of people.

However, today, especially in the last 200 years, we have modern processed foods in abundance. These tend to be high in the glycemic index. They include any kind of processed sugar or grain, including rice and wheat. Likely most overweight people eat these foods and get the large insulin blood sugar spike. Insulin turns on the body engine to store extra energy as fat, and then the body crashes after the meal because the high glycemic foods are quick to digest.

So this type of person gets hungry again quickly. This cycle continues onward and a person of that 25% high glycemic insulin reaction group tends to be overweight and always hungry.

To deal with this problem such a person can choose foods that are natural and healthy with a lower rating in glycemic index. This is not to say they can never have the higher glycemic index foods, but should at least mix these with lower glycemic index foods. Also eating a meal with healthy fat and protein along with carbohydrates in proper proportion tends to slow down the insulin response to the high glycemic index foods. Another technique is to add in lemon juice or apple cider vinegar to the meal. This will also slow down the insulin response.

In ancient human history, most people ate a diet made up of lower glycemic index carbohydrates. Therefore, the body is not used to a high carbohydrate diet with so many high glycemic index foods. When man started farming grains, this started to add in extra carbohydrate energy into the diet. This is good for civilization, because it enabled storing up of foods for the winter.

Nevertheless, in recent times we went too far with processed foods and sugary foods. Modern civilization raised the glycemic index up too high in the foods that are eaten. At the same time, these energy dense foods became too easily available and exercise levels dropped due to mechanization.

Today we are having generations of fat unhealthy people. Genetically it seems to be the luck of the draw of how your body reacts to high glycemic foods. If your part of the lucky 25% you tend to be thin. However, realize even this lucky thin 25% can be unhealthy due to lack of good nutrition.

At this point, you may want to reflect, do I tend to be overweight? What about my family, are they overweight as well? What is my family history with diabetes? Do I eat excess carbohydrates, especially the processed carbohydrates? Do I crave carbohydrates? How can I tell my reaction to a high glycemic index meal? If I eat a large high glycemic meal, do I feel somewhat high for a while, and then get sleepy afterward and need a nap? If so, this may be because of the high insulin response and the crash afterward due to the lack of blood sugar to the brain. This reaction may increase, as you get older.

The solution is simple, concentrate on eating low glycemic index foods. This will help get blood sugar stabilized over the whole day. You will store less body fat because you will not eat so much food in-between meals.

A short practical list of high index foods is white rice, white potatoes, sugary foods and drinks and processed grain products such as breads, cakes and cookies. As a rule, any grain that is processed is a higher glycemic index item.

Avoid or limit sweetened foods and drinks. Avoid anything not natural, and made by processing with sugars or carbohydrates. It is an unhealthy higher glycemic item.

These considerations depend on your physical condition and genetics as well. You need more care if you are diabetic and overweight than if you are thinner in shape and not diabetic. Also, consider family history and age. For instance if you are healthy today, young, thin and active, that is good. However, if your family history is to have diabetes, you have an opportunity to prevent that future condition or make it less severe.

Replace high glycemic foods with natural fruits and vegetables. For example if you make brown rice spaghetti, this is a fine food with a medium glycemic index number, but the bulk of the meal should be vegetables with some oil and protein. Same thing with white rice and white potatoes, these are fine foods. However, limit the portions and have a large amount of low glycemic index foods such as vegetables.

I love bread, (typically, a high glycemic index food) but I have found that most store bought breads affect me negatively. Sadly, modern processing of bread has taken it far away from the natural bread of older times. Oddball fats, excessive yeasts, additives and so on are in use in modern bread making. If you desire bread, look for the most natural whole-wheat or sourdough breads that you can find. Sourdough breads use natural yeast in processing. It is a slower method of bread making not popular for manufacturing. Modern sourdough bread can have food additives as well, so seek out the most natural kinds.

Many types of modern store breads indicate on packaging they are natural and healthy, but may have processing that is harmful. As a practical manner, it is difficult for me to tell by feeling my body the positive effects when abstaining from store bought breads. However, I can tell over a long time a positive result, such as weeks to months. Many people think they have a negative reaction to gluten when eating bread products, but it may be from other causes such as excessive yeast or food additives.

For health, instead of commercially made bread, eat rice or potatoes. Instead of a prepackaged meal, make a pot of steamed vegetables. Instead of opening a can of common premade sauce, try the organic versions or a can of organic peeled whole tomatoes. In other words, try to change your daily eating habits as far as you can toward the least processed foods. The ultimate is eating only organic foods in a natural form, lightly cooked, not canned or frozen and in season, buying organic or growing organic. As a practical manner, this ideal is not possible for most of us, but be as close as you can. I personally think the healthiest forms of canned and frozen foods to be acceptable, frozen to be better than canned.

We all have different genetics and family histories. There is no blanket recommendation for everyone on what to eat and in what proportion. Consider your own family history and experiment on how you feel as you work on your program. In all cases, everyone should be striving for the least processed healthy foods. This means home cooking using source foods.

For snacking, consider eating raw nuts and seeds along with raw vegetables and fruits. When dieting raw vegetables and fruits are a good choice, while remembering nuts and seeds are high in fat, so should be limited.

Chapter Six

How to eat considering personal genetics and exercise

Personal genetics will determine somewhat what is good to eat. Let us consider some different situations. A common one is a person who wants to lose weight; and they are part of the 25% human population who has a large insulin reaction to high glycemic index foods.

In that case, he or she wants to reduce the high glycemic index foods in their diet, selecting the right kinds of foods to help extend the time in-between meals. Remember any extra eaten fat is easily stored as body fat, so they want a minimum fat intake, but still need essential fats in their daily diet. The body cannot make essential fatty acids such as the Omega 3's or Omega 6's.

They would eat olive oil, flax oil, nuts, seeds, olives and any other healthy sources of fat. They would be strictly against any unhealthy fat, such as from saturated fat sources, limiting unhealthy margarine spreads, lard, ice cream and fatty red meats.

They should eat most kinds of fruits and vegetables raw or lightly cooked. It takes more energy and time to convert these low glycemic index carbohydrates to body fat than the high glycemic carbohydrates or fats. Therefore, this helps to extend the time in-between meals. In reality to lose weight, a person must take in fewer calories than what they use to and most people will feel a little hungry while losing weight. Therefore, it really helps to get a nice full feeling at mealtime. Eating a low glycemic meal will last longer with a fuller feeling until the next meal.

Another example, let us say you are part of the thin 25% of the human spectrum. You have a low insulin reaction to carbohydrates and do not put on the body fat. In this case, you do not need to lose weight; in fact, you may want to gain weight. Excess fat in the diet will easily convert to body weight so you may want to increase healthy fat intake, and still eat mostly nutritious lower glycemic foods. However, eating low glycemic is not as important for a thin person as for an overweight person with their higher insulin reaction. Remember, even though you may have a lower insulin reaction to high glycemic foods, you still can get diabetes and other illnesses in time by eating too much high glycemic index junk foods.

I personally know someone who worked construction all his life. He is tough and thin, but he drank soda pops every day for many years. Now he has diabetes and is much reduced in strength. He is still mentally tough, but his body is a broken shell of what it was and what it could be today-if he kept his health.

A person can be thin and still be unhealthy because of poor lifestyle. For instance, take a jogger who has a major heart attack. A likely cause is bad food. If he or she ate too many processed foods with additives, this will clog arteries. If you feel any kind of chest pain or congestion, and have high blood pressure (nosebleeds), be sure to clean up your diet no matter your weight or physical condition. See a health care provider, your life may depend on it.

Observe your loved ones. Do they have chest pains? Such pains can go on for years and they may say little or nothing, then a heart attack. It is time to clean up the diet, only the absolute best effort may work. Most should take the pills the doctor recommends, especially if not serious about a clean diet. If one treats clogged arteries with diet alone, you must be strict. Stricter than most can imagine, no cheating, *just a little cheating* with bad processed foods will undo all other effort. A strict clean diet must be followed for the rest of life.

Another example: let us say you are a weight lifter. In this instance, you will need more protein and likely to take protein supplementation. If so, monitor how your kidneys feel, and consider choosing the cleanest natural protein sources over supplements. For example beans, eggs or egg whites, a few raw nuts, seeds and lastly clean meat. Depending on your body type and genetics, thin or heavy, these will indicate your fat intake while sticking to the healthiest fats. Feel your body, do not over eat protein and give your muscles time to heal. This practice will help avoid overtaxing your organs.

All people should eat more of the lower glycemic index carbohydrates no matter their body type. Some thin people may be a little less careful if they choose to and not get fat, but even they can become sickly over time.

There can be times when a person may want a higher glycemic index food. For instance, after a hard workout and needing a quick recovery. If so, you may eat a higher glycemic food such as bananas with a sports drink to help muscles and liver regain carbohydrate energy. However, if you are of the 25% group with a high insulin reaction to carbohydrates, you need to be careful with this practice.

How do you tell if your part of the high insulin reaction group? See a health care professional for testing. Otherwise, indicators are body type and family history. Is your family full of overweight people with diabetes? If so, then it is more likely. When you eat excess sugar and high glycemic index carbohydrates, do you get a sugar high, crash later on, and eat excessively? These are possible indicators.

Let us imagine you are a runner or a mountain climber. After a hard run or mountain climb you may want a little extra protein so you eat beans, seeds and nuts. In addition, you feel dragged down, so you eat some high glycemic foods such as bananas and potatoes to get your muscles back full of energy quickly. You really burned the calories during the run or climb so you do not worry about any extra fat intake. In fact, you may want to take in extra Omega 3 fatty acids before and after the big event because they are anti-inflammatory. One can take a tablespoon of flaxseed oil, which is naturally high in omega 3 fatty acids, instead of taking over the counter anti-inflammatory painkillers. You rest up a few days before the next big event.

Alternatively, if the next exercise event is very soon, maybe the next day. You take in a lot of easy to digest high glycemic carbohydrates to refill carbohydrate energy stores in the muscles, liver and intestines. In addition, you eat some slow digesting low glycemic foods with fats to get you through a long race or climb.

For example, at first, eat fast digesting high glycemic index foods such as bananas, white bread, white rice, white potatoes, pretzels, rice bread, and rice cakes. Add in some salt and electrolytes-maybe a sports drink to wash it down. After this, eat some slower digesting mid-range to low-range glycemic foods, such as whole grain breads, cooked whole grains, fruits, and vegetables. For protein, consider eating beans, nuts, and seeds being careful not to bog down the digestion system. Thinking along these lines, you can intelligently prepare for another strenuous event coming up soon.

The variations of what to eat depend on what your body needs, the kind of exercise and time until the next event.

Do you need fat for a low intensity, slow breathing exercise like hiking, or is it a sprint? How far off is the next event? If it is in a few minutes, eat a little of the fastest digesting high glycemic foods that you can handle. Is it in a few hours or longer away? Then fill up on easy digesting high glycemic foods and low glycemic foods in a combination suited to the kind of exercise coming up.

In marathons, runners often hit a lack of energy wall because they run out of stored carbohydrates. This often happens around 22 miles, because they exhausted their store of energy in muscles and liver. To help prevent this, runners eat or drink easy to digest high glycemic carbohydrates during the race. In addition, mountain climbers may eat high glycemic foods during a long climb. They want something sugary; maybe raw honey with a little fat from flax seed oil-put these in a squeeze tube and add a touch of sea salt. There are sugary sports products such as sports drinks and goo's that are available. These provide quick energy along with electrolytes (salts and minerals in solution; such as sodium, potassium, calcium and magnesium) to prevent cramps.

Remember raw nuts, seeds and greens along with other natural foods are a great daily source of electrolytes (mineral salts when in solution). These are easy on the digestion system in comparison to concentrated supplements.

If you are hiking with a slow breathing rate, you tend to be burning body fat, if you are breathing hard you are using more carbohydrates. Sometimes your breathing is varied and you are using both kinds of body fuel. It is a matter of proportions; most exercises use both kinds of energy.

For more endurance set your pace to breathe easy when working or walking. When hiking I try to set my pace to be breathing easy in order to burn mostly fat and save my carbohydrate energy. Some people like to hike with a fast breathing rate and rest at intervals. This method burns more carbohydrate energy.

Chapter Seven

Understanding an initial health diet

I concentrate primarily on a health diet, not a lose weight diet. However, if you follow a healthy eating program and eat two meals a day, one can lose weight. The way to lose weight and keep it off is not a fad diet program, but to have a long-term lifestyle change. What your new lifestyle will be is up to you. It can be difficult to come up with a long-term positive lifestyle in this hectic world, but with determination it is something you can control.

There are many different paths toward good health, a person should have a healthy diet and not overeat in a maintainable lifestyle. The best kind of program is a positive lifestyle habit, with enough variations to prevent boredom. Every person should consciously decide on his or her lifestyle, I give my ideas and experiences as well as Biblical Daniel's in this book. In addition, you should study other information sources. In all this information and thought will be your lifestyle program. Talk to God about what to do and he will help with mental impressions.

Many people have a "sick cow syndrome" because they eat too many empty calories. An example is the person with dull cow like eyes who waddles into the fast food joint and eats bad foods. They fatten up with unhealthy food, and then waddle out. Soon enough they are hungry again for unhealthier high calorie foods.

They are over fed in calories and under nourished, and probably are craving nutrition and not getting it. Does this person need more calories with empty nutrition? No, what they need is less calories and more nutrition. However, they are in a trap, their body chemistry is adapted to this bad diet and they are mentally hooked to it. They do not feel good unless they are eating in this way. They are craving excess fats, sugars, carbohydrates, salts, and even meat.

Often people physically crave what is not good for them and this can include chocolate, caffeine, high glycemic carbohydrates and more. This can be because of food addiction. If you think you have a food addiction, then study this subject and see a naturopathic or ecological doctor. Some symptoms of food addiction are craving a food item, being high after ingesting and afterward having a crash. In addition, if you do not ingest the suspected food or drink, you have withdrawal symptoms and feel unwell. These symptoms may increase as you get older.

Are you hooked on an unhealthy eating pattern? Is this you? This condition can be at differing levels, from mild to extreme. To go from a poor lifestyle to a healthier one needs a transition time for most people. Most people would fail a sudden strict Biblical Daniel's diet and lifestyle. Most of us cannot do it all at once, but still want to change for the better. Anyone can do it in small steps of transition toward better diet and lifestyle.

Steps in transition means you select small

things to change for the better, like giving up coffee for herbal teas. You can change a diet of eating excessive meat to one with less meat in steps.

For each change wait until feeling solid with it before going to next positive lifestyle change or experiment. How long it takes for each change varies for the individual. It may take several days or a week, a month, even longer, no matter be patient with yourself. I suggest giving up coffee and replacing it with herbal tea, take a week or a month to get it solid. Then work on another diet or lifestyle change item next month and so on. I find this to be a never-ending process for me as I experiment with diet, exercise and lifestyle to see if something else is better.

I also try out new things to prevent boredom in life, being careful not to make mistakes by monitoring my body closely and studying broadly. Note, it is possible to damage yourself before you know it with conventional or alternative products that are said to be good for health. As a rule, I shy away from manmade items that are not natural or exotic to my body. I am cautious about anything said to have a powerful effect.

Any new diet and lifestyle will be your achievement. You will choose it yourself to meet your needs. Are you excited? I am, I believe in you! God will help you! I do not think there is one exact best diet or lifestyle, which will work for everyone, although there are similarities in most good health programs. I strongly encourage you to read many books on the subject of health and lifestyle. I find that various health experts tend to have their own main area of focus and core beliefs, and these are different from one expert to another. However, all the good experts are similar to each other. To get a balanced view it is necessary to obtain information from many sources.

Beware; some health information sources have a non-honest agenda. If you chose to ingest unhealthy items in excess and think it healthy because of a biased information source you will suffer for it. For myself, I limit or avoid, cheese, chocolate, dairy, caffeine, altered oils, GMO corn products and more. There are information sources that say these are good for you and information sources that say they are suspect. Often what people believe to be true is according to their personality, rather than intelligence.

There are biased information sources both ways. What is the truth? That can be difficult to tell. Use how you feel as a primary guide and be honest. Do you feel an adverse effect? Do you feel an excessively strong effect that is unnatural feeling? Do you get high off chocolate and caffeine or something else and then feel down afterward. Alternatively, do you feel bad if you cannot get it? If so, that strong effect may be an indication to avoid or limit something. Finding independent experts that you trust are a method to help figure out what is safe. However, always use how you feel is the final guide.

I have a strong inclination to follow Biblical Daniel in diet and limit supplements and pills of any kind, even medicinal herbs. I concentrate on ingesting healthy foods and drinks for medicine and nutrition. I have tried in the past a semi healthy diet with many supplements with moderate to poor results. Today, I have a diet as close to Biblical Daniels that I can, with a decent lifestyle. I find that I am healthier with the pulse foods diet and eating two meals a day with few supplements. I am always experimenting, but in a careful way.

Be cautious of scientific studies, as the study may have an intentional bias for some desired result, many studies are paid for by commercial industry. Industry pays for most studies that are used by the government to judge the safety of a new product. Often the real study happens when the product is in use by the public. Therefore, I am very cautious about new products of any kind such as medications, supplements, GMO, food additives, herbicides and pesticides. Even honest studies that are positive for a short time may not indicate long-term bad effects.

Even be careful of honest health experts. They can make mistakes because it may take a long time for undesirable effects to be noticeable in personal experience. Experts are people too and everyone has different genetics, and family history, therefore everyone reacts differently. Sometimes ill effects from mistakes are hard or impossible to reverse. Think about diet and lifestyle over supplementation and pill taking while working toward better health.

I have a friend who took colloidal silver for health. Unfortunately, this silver had high nitric acid (HNO3) content; the acid seriously damaged his teeth. He said his fillings would decay and fall out, and that this happened over several weeks while he was taking it. Sadly, he did not figure out the cause before it was too late. A high voltage arc makes this type of colloidal silver. Correctly, made colloidal silver does not have this acid. Well-made colloidal silver used correctly can be beneficial. The lesson here is to be very careful of supplementation, and to do research before taking anything, to watch very closely the effects, good or bad. It is possible to have damage before you know it, especially if not monitoring carefully.

If a person will pay attention to how their body feels when doing experimentation, they will know the truth in time. In studying various health programs, be careful of extremes. Like a long-term only raw foods diet, or a medical approach that discounts diet concerns. Often information sources contradict each other. If so, do additional study. I don't want to discourage you in experimentation, but be cautious about claims. In money and health if it is too good to be true, then it is likely a fraud. I favor natural gentle ways in diet and supplementation while avoiding extremes.

More about transition, on how to go toward better diet and lifestyle

If you want to be more like Biblical Daniel, and less like King Nebuchadnezzar, great! You are ready to begin! Here is how you can do it. Instead of changing all bad eating habits at once, change one thing at a time. Wait for about a week or two for each change to stabilize and then change something else. If you need a longer time, this is fine. If you can do changes quicker, even better.

For example, I gave up coffee and soda pop. I replaced coffee with jasmine green tea, and later on, I went to herbal teas. I then replaced soda pop with fruit juice. I did each change for about a week without any other changes. After I had the coffee and soda pop under control, I began to make other changes. I gave up most dairy products and this was easy for me. I replaced dairy with rice and soymilk products. Then after a very long time, I reduced my dairy milk replacements close to zero.

Not everyone needs to reduce cow's milk products to zero it depends on genetics. Some people may be able to eat yogurt and cottage cheese and other products made from dairy because they have less lactose. It depends on the person, as to how much they can digest without ill effect. Each person has his or her own amount of lactase, the enzyme that digests milk sugar lactose. When people get older, most have less amounts of lactase. Watch how you feel carefully, as you may have a slight negative effect to lactose that will harm health and be hard to detect. An acute adverse reaction to lactose or casein (milk protein) may cause phlegm in the throat (excessive throat clearing) and or digestive problems.

Remember, even if you can digest dairy fine, non-organic dairy may have hormones, antibiotics and other toxins in trace amounts. Excess hormones in children's diet from animal products can have undesirable results.

After a few months, I began to concentrate

on wheat products. I limit all wheat-based products including whole wheat. I replaced these with rice-based products and other whole grain products. The reason I gave up the wheat-based products is the gluten content, which is an allergen source. It can tend to glue up the intestines in some people. However, natural whole grain breads made similar to those made during Biblical times are better for health. The modern fine grain products are more suspect. It is possible to find coarse whole-wheat products made in an older traditional way that is healthier. Look for local bakeries that make the better breads.

Did you know glue could be made from white flour to glue on wallpaper! It is because of the gluten in the flour. This practice was common in the old days when people put up new wallpaper every spring. You may not need to give up all suspicious bad food products such as gluten. However, in your personal experimenting you can remove and carefully add back foods to see how you feel. Be aware there can be slight bad reactions that are hard to tell and will slowly erode health in time.

I personally find that eating large amounts of modern processed wheat products causes brain fog and bloating while digesting. Such affects may go un-noticed by most people. They are either non-affected or the effect is slight. It is likely many people are affected to some degree, but unable to tell until older when the effect increases. Meanwhile over the years, this has sapped health.

I often speak to people who say they have

no problem with wheat or other common allergen foods, but I wonder. One way to test most anything is totally remove it from the diet for about two weeks and then eat a large amount of it. Be careful if you are allergic, it may cause a bad reaction.

In my personal experience, I could not feel the effects from processed wheat products until I changed my diet to a cleaner one and only then, I could tell. Today, if I eat white wheat pasta it feels like a large lump in my belly and it hurts my intestines. However, years before I ate it with no thought.

I gave up the common unhealthy sugary fatty treats, such ice cream, cakes, pastries and cookies. I replaced these with similar healthier items from the health food store by reading and comparing the food labels. After a long time, I reduced even these healthier items close to zero. Still today, I may have an urge to binge eat and if so, I go for the more healthy options. It is best to keep unhealthy treats out of the house to avoid cheating. Honestly, I still struggle time to time with tasty snacks. It helps to have a goal to work toward to stay on track.

Limit fat laden grain fed meats. Instead, eat free-range lean meat that is grass fed. Look for chicken and turkey that are free range. Free-range means naturally fed animals, which means leaner better meat. Nothing deep-fried is healthy. The high temperature during frying changes the molecular structure of the fat to something unhealthy.

In my meat eating transitioning, at first I ate

cleaner meat as often as I needed, and I slowly reduced the amount and ate more fish, vegetable and nut based proteins. One can go to zero meat if you prefer, like Biblical Daniel. I do not see a big difference between zero meat and a little clean meat for long-term health. The key here is eating *very small amounts* of clean meat for health. The absolute best may be zero meat for long-term health, but it is up to the individual.

Exactly how each person decides to eat meat is a personal choice. Just understand the principles. If you have a family history of heart disease, then you may want to be stricter with unclean fatty red meats. If there is little family history of heart disease, then you may be a little more liberal. Remember, Biblical Daniel would hardly ever eat meat. Certainly, he ate none during his trial and learning years. I personally feel the best when I eat meat less than once a week.

I am conscious of eating protein in balance; meat by itself is a balanced protein. For vegetarians there can be a concern about obtaining enough B vitamins, especially B12. I use nutritional yeast when preparing food to get plenty of B vitamins. Beans and rice are a balanced protein-I often eat these together. You can eat raw nuts, seeds, and eggs, some health experts say to limit nuts and seeds to handful or so day. I think the reason for this advice is to avoid developing a food allergy to nuts and seeds.

I had two adverse reactions to eating excessive nuts in my life. In my early thirties, I was eating in excess roasted nuts for protein and my prostate started to hurt. It took me two months to figure out why. This pain went away when I stopped eating the roasted nuts (The large pile of supplements that I tried did not cure me). The roasting of the nuts changes the molecular structure of the oil in the nut to something less healthy. This altered oil is what hurt my prostate.

The second instance is many years later. I started to eat a mixture of raw nuts; I ate too much for several months and started to get a skin rash on my belly. Once again, it took a couple of months for me to figure out the cause. That it was a nut allergy; it went away when I reduced my intake of raw nuts and seeds. So eating raw nuts and seeds is good, but not in excess. In general, small handfuls of each kind a day is best, and see how it goes for you.

I personally find eggs to be a great protein source, but they are easy to overeat. When I do so, they increase my cholesterol and blood pressure. For others it may depend on genetics. One can gain a food addiction relationship to eggs and have an allergy, especially if you eat in excess.

Many health sources say it is best to limit eggs to around four a week. Although I know of someone who eats about three eggs every morning and he is healthy. However, he works in construction and burns it off. If you experiment with egg count, try to feel how your heart is doing, how congested it feels. If you pay attention, it may be possible to feel high blood pressure by feeling the blood pressure in your head and body. Nosebleeds are a possible sign of high blood pressure. Better yet, buy a blood pressure measuring device from the drug store. It is advisable if you are thirties and older to get your blood pressure and cholesterol checked, especially if overweight.

I often feel heart congestion if I eat excess processed foods with hydrogenated oil or any other modified oil. I get the same feeling with eggs if I eat too many over a time. I get a congested feeling in my chest and heart circulatory system. I notice that the organic brown eggs are richer and they seem to have a more powerful thickening effect on my blood and heart circulatory system. This is only my subjective personal experience.

Excess protein is hard on the kidneys and kidney damage may sneak up on you. If you overdo protein in youth, you may pay for it by poor kidney health later on in life. I myself find it best not to use protein powders, because it is a strain on my kidneys, especially now that I am in my forties. In my younger years, I felt no ill effect when I used protein powders on occasion.

Kidney pain is different from spinal back pain, but it is easy to confuse spinal back pain with kidney pain as they are close together in the same area of the body. The kidneys are located along the sides of the backbone right over the hips in the back. If you are mind-body aware, you will know where the pain is coming from. Although it may be difficult when you have both pains blended in together. If so, you must be careful and find the exact source of the pain for treatment.

A common example is the person with a small amount of chronic lower back pain, and then the overall back pain gets much worse due to kidney pain. If the person thinks the new kidney pain is from the spinal area or pulled muscles, then treatment will be incorrect. The most common cause of kidney pain is some sort of toxin that the person is ingesting, such as excess protein, tea, coffee, supplements, vitamins etc. For people with sensitive kidneys the pain may come on quickly or slowly. For instance, it may take a few days due to something new in the diet. On the other hand, it can come on over a long time due to an adverse food or beverage item, such as excessive coffee.

If you eat a lot of meat, your body is adapted to this eating pattern and it may be difficult to go quickly to a limited amount of meat, (I remember this situation for myself long ago). If you find yourself in this situation, it is ok, just come up with a plan of transition toward eating less meat. There is no single perfect way of being healthy and becoming healthier. We all find our own paths, the key is to be aware and work on a plan of action. Eat the cleaner meats in lesser amounts at each sitting and slowly reduce to what you think is optimum to eat each month.

It is possible to eat fresh clean meat with its fat as a primary diet item, because Eskimos do so in their traditional diet. In today's modern world, urban people do not get clean fresh meat like the traditional Eskimo. For most people I think its best to limit meat intake for the longest healthy lifespan.

I initially would crave meat when I started

limiting meat intake. My body was used to eating more meat than what I now considered the optimum. I slowly reduced how often I ate meat, and I ate more beans and nuts and my body adapted to the new diet. If you are in this situation, take time and work a transition. For me, it took longer than a year to transition to where I wanted to be in meat eating.

The same could be for any kind of food or beverage. The body chemistry can be used to an unhealthy diet that can take a long time to change. In addition, the body can be craving an allergen causing food or beverage. One item that I lust for sometimes is chocolate, and I indulge more often than I should. My favorite is chocolate chip cookies and I often pay for it. What is your weakness?

One rule I had in the beginning days of transitioning, is that I do not care how much the better foods cost, or how much I eat, as long it is a healthier alternative. This can be your rule as well.

All of us have crutches or habits we use when dealing with stress. One common way of dealing with stress is to eat a lot of junk food. If this is you, it can be dealt with. You may eat as much as you want during the transitioning phases toward better diet habits. Nevertheless, you should follow some rules you lay down for yourself. I suggest that you substitute your un-healthy binge foods with better alternatives from the health food store, and binge away. I speak from experience. A couple of boxes of non-wheat organic chocolate chip cookies on occasion when stressed out will not destroy your diet.

People respond to stress in different ways, I am a stress eater, so when I stress-I eat. Some people are the opposite, they stress and will not eat. If you are a stress eater, choose the healthiest items you can find to indulge. Afterward, when you are full, bloated and feeling sick, you can vow to get back on track with your health program tomorrow. Since you ate the healthier items, mentally you stayed on *your* program.

For example at night, I may indulge in a massive bowl of fruit topped with soy or rice ice cream! If you need to do this for a period, weeks to months, even longer, do so. Later on, you can consider not having after dinner snacking, but at first, it is not that important. The most important thing at first is eating better foods. After this is solid you can work on controlling the times and amounts of food eaten.

It is a common situation, that you start a lifestyle improvement program, but you are used to eating a lot of meat, sugars, processed carbohydrates, saturated fats, drinking coffee and also chocolates etc. You have been overweight and out of shape for the last few years. Now is the time to do something. You remember a happy active youth; you were thinner, felt better and looked better.

You may want to resolve to go toward a better lifestyle, no matter how long it takes. Just do small steps, as you need. Give up coffee this week or this month, replace it with herbal teas, and get that under your belt, then go to the next bad item of lifestyle, exercise, food or beverage to work on.

For example you may still eat meat too often, but look for the more healthy alternatives, slowly reducing the portions of meat and how often. Instead of deep-fried, choose baked meat, in smaller proportions, and then try home cooked free-range fed meat. At the same time, replace the less healthy versions of chocolate with more healthy versions of dark organic chocolate. Think about health transitioning in this way.

After a few weeks to months of transitioning, your eating pattern will be much better than before. You are conscious of what you are eating and making intelligent choices. You are reading many sources of health information, and looking at food labels. You are now on the right path, on a personal quest for best health!

A side benefit of a cleaner diet is that you will have less body odor and smell in the armpit region. It is because a person with a cleaner diet will have fewer toxins to remove. Overall health and strength is better, up to ten times higher than before.

For most people only after having a better eating pattern on solid ground is it time to think about losing weight. To get to that point may take a long time, possibly up to a year or longer.

We are ready to think about a 10-day diet test program

The strict program is only eating Pulse foods for ten days-that means avoiding meat for ten days. What are the Pulse foods? They are fruits, vegetables, coarse natural grains, seeds and nuts.

Fruits are apples, bananas, oranges, mangos, watermelon, cantaloupe, pineapple and more.

Vegetables are broccoli, spinach, cabbage, tomato, potato, sweet potato, seaweed and beans, and more.

The raw nuts or seeds are pecans, walnuts, cashews, sunflower seeds, pumpkin seeds, flax seeds, chia seeds, sesame seeds and more.

The staple grains in our house are rice and oats. There are many other good grains as well. Grains are seeds that need to be cooked to be eaten. If you have trouble digesting grains or seeds, it is possible to soak them, or sprout them to be easier to digest.

You need a source of healthy fats. Restricting fat too much is a common mistake when trying to lose weight and getting healthier. People need to eat fat or oil, so should have it in the diet. If you stop eating fat the body will revolt in time. In desperation, you will crash back into old bad eating patterns to get the fat you need.

Plan on a healthy fat intake source; if you need take a tablespoon or two of flaxseed oil a day and put olive oil in food. When trying to lose weight it is important not to over eat fat and high glycemic index carbohydrates, but you need some fat.

My staple fat sources are olive oil in food and flax seed oil for supplementation, but there are other healthy oils. We use safflower oil and grape seed oil for higher temperature cooking. I like olive oil and walnut oil for lower temperature cooking and on salads.

The major aim of transition toward a health diet is not losing weight, but to change eating patterns toward a healthier way. Only afterward, if you desire, think about losing weight. When that will be is up to you. You do not want a plan doomed to fail, by dieting too soon and falling back into past bad eating habits. A healthier eating habit will stick with you no matter if you lose weight or not.

I know from personal experience that you can eat healthy foods in excess and not lose weight. So eating in a healthier way may not by itself help you lose weight. No matter, you can transition yourself to where you want to be in time.

My personal example is when I first married; the wife and my eating patterns were different. I happily ate a bunch of smaller meals in a day, but she is used to two to three larger meals a day. So the first few years of marriage I would eat my smaller meals AND the larger meals. She was a social eater so I had to eat with her for a happy home life and of course, I was accustomed to cleaning off my plate.

I did not get extremely fat, but I went from 180lbs to 220lbs eating healthy foods before I figured out what was going on. I ate three full meals a day and added in my accustomed snacks. In addition, I was getting older and my metabolism was slowing down. I was stacking food on top of food in my belly with no rest for my digestion system. I was putting in new food before the old food digested.

My eating background was so different from my wife's that something had to change. At first, I decided to eat less in general and I lost down to 195lbs, but I never could get rid of that extra fifteen pounds. In the last year, I went to two meals a day with rare snacking midday. Lately my weight is around 186 with no real effort. All my clothes are fitting looser these days.

Two meals a day is a lifestyle change that took me a long time to get mentally ready to try. The two meals a day program is an old way to restrict excess food intake for people who do light to moderate levels of work. In any health habit, it is best to have daily lifestyle patterns to keep, such as two meals a day. It is more difficult to maintain weight without structure because you may find yourself eating all the time!

It took me a long time to be mentally ready for a two meals a day diet program, so do not rush. It may take you a year and longer if you are coming from an unhealthy lifestyle. An alternative is a many meals a day diet program, but you will need to count calories to lose weight. In all diet programs, I think for best health it is good to stop eating food after the evening meal-to let the digestion organs clean out food until morning.

When you are ready for two meals a day diet program, it will get the weight off and keep it off *for the rest of your life.*

Chapter Eight
Losing weight by lifestyle change

A fully formed adult needs fewer calories, but often people keep eating like a teenager when they get older. Many people are accustomed to three meals a day and finishing off full plates of food. Then having snacks whenever a slight hunger pang hits due to a nervous twitch, this is a fattening habit- especially when older.

If you are disciplined and if it is important for you to lose weight, the method I recommend is eating two meals a day. The only allowed midday snacks are raw fruit, raw vegetables, raw seeds and raw nuts, all in a plain form. The evening meal should be no later than 6pm on average. There should be no snacking after the evening meal. Less strict is an occasional glass of fruit juice or a piece of fruit or something else similarly light after the evening meal.

Eat two balanced healthy meals every day, with good nutrition and eat until full, do not overeat or under eat. With exercise, this will get you to the correct body weight in time, it can take many months to a year or longer. It is important to have two balanced meals. Only an adult doing hard labor or a growing child needs more than two good meals a day. As an alternative, you can eat a slightly more substantial snack lunch mid-day at work, but it will be harder to lose weight.

Healthy balanced meals mean you have

healthy forms of carbohydrates, sugars, fats and proteins in your meals. You must do some meal planning, because if you miss one or more meals you are not getting balanced nutrition. For instance, you can have beans and rice for carbohydrates and protein, then put some olive oil in the food for fat. The olive oil can be in a dollop of veganaise on top of the beans or cooked in with the rice.

If your current weight is fine and you are not eating late at night, then most likely whatever eating pattern you already have is good, no need to change.

Why only two meals a day?

It is simple, you do not have to worry about counting calories, and it is difficult, almost impossible to overeat with two meals a day. The mid-day snack is only to help you through this hunger point. If you really want to lose weight, stop the snack and be strict with the two meals a day. Meals moderate to large, and eat until full every time, but do not gorge.

Another benefit of two meals a day is it lets your digestion system rest. The long period between the second meal and breakfast lets, your organs clean out. Therefore, the body can concentrate on healing, rather than endlessly digesting.

Understand an overeating condition that many people have. A person eats a meal or snack then afterward, too soon is another meal, then another. They are stacking food on top of food-on top of food, etc. This is more likely if overweight; a common condition is people over eating due to stress. It is nervous eating; not eating because of hunger. For some people the mental and physical response to stress is eating. In addition, it can be a habit to overeat, such as eating three full meals a day; this is too much food for most people.

If you find yourself pushing out food from the intestines, before it has time to digest, you are *extremely* overeating. To get control over this situation is by understanding the overeating. If it is due to stress then find positive ways to deal with the stress. If it is due to a daily overeating habit, work on changing the habit.

For long-term health, the two meals a day program is hard to beat. A many meals a day diet program depends on limiting each meal size and it is easy to start slipping up. The two meals a day program is a lifelong lifestyle change. If you eat more than two meals, you know instantly, you are off the program. If you are snacking with the wrong foods, you know you are off the program.

In the beginning of eating only two meals a day, you may need to stuff yourself at meal times. However, unless you are doing hard physical work, you do not need to eat to an extreme. Therefore, in about a month, you will get used to this eating schedule and eat less each meal.

If you need more food for hard physical work, you can increase your mid-day snack as long as you need. While understanding that this is not permanent after the hard working period ends. Adults need to be careful when restricting children's eating habits, most children need more than two meals a day as they are growing and very active. It is difficult for a child to eat enough food in two meals, because their bellies are smaller. Fully formed adults are in a different situation; they have less activity, not growing, and have a slower metabolism.

It may be difficult to follow a strict two meals a day program with an unstable schedule. It works best if your lifestyle and work situation is regular. Nevertheless, for most people, when eating more than two meals a day it is easy to overeat. Therefore, calories need to be counted out to prevent this.

I sometimes find two meals a day are fine until my schedule gets too hectic. I then find it difficult to get in my second meal at a good time. Therefore, I make compromises. Such as a small snack to get through to the evening meal, a single apple works very well.

While working, plan your snack "lunch" to stay on the program. The lunch should consist mostly of raw vegetables and fruit, with a little of raw nuts and seeds. This is a snack; therefore, you do not worry about eating a balanced meal.

Social demands from other people can make it difficult to maintain a health diet while visiting friends or family. Eating is a social function that is hard to get out of without hurting feelings. I cheat a little at such social functions, once a week or so off the plan will not kill a two meals a day program. If a known social meal is coming up, you can eat the morning meal and the needed snack to get by. Then wait until the social function to have the second meal at whatever time it happens. Even with a hectic lifestyle, the program is working fine. I am at my proper weight and feeling great.

Another method is if I need to eat a larger mid-day snack because of a hectic day pushing my second meal way out late. I just reduce the last meal in size and this is a good compromise. It is a common notion that the biggest meal of the day must be breakfast. I do not agree, I think eating so much food in the morning may make a person feel bloated and ill all morning, especially if doing physical labor. My larger meal is in the evening after work, which is better for me. To lose weight it is best to have no late night snacking after the last meal. A lifelong lifestyle to keep weight off is no snacking after the evening meal. Less effective is light snacking after the evening meal.

A suggested program to lose weight is to pick a reasonable target weight. If you can, tie this target weight goal into another goal, such as looking good in a bathing suit or doing a hiking trip. Then eat two meals a day with little to zero snacking. Eat two complete healthy meals and exercise. Eat like this until you reach your target weight then evaluate. If you can eat light snacking mid-day without gaining weight, then do so. However, if weight starts to go back up above the target, instantly go back to a strict two meals a day, in this way you can maintain weight. If you still eat too much food with two cooked meals, you can choose to eat a pure raw foods meal for one of the meals. The weight should come off slowly with such a program.

If you eat only two meals a day, I found in a couple of weeks my stomach will shrink and I tend to eat less. However, at first I was extremely hungry and wanted to stuff myself. In time, this lessened. Go with the flow. Eat until full at the two meal times. Most people will lose weight and keep it off for the rest of their lifespan with this practice. Experiment and do what is best for you.

Some people may find eating a large volume of food that is low in calories for a midday snack to work better for them. *If you do this, this must be of extremely low calorie natural foods, meaning no fats and sugars.* Eat only raw or lightly cooked fruits and vegetables in a plain form. Very little to zero dried fruits or nuts and seeds, the key here is very low calorie natural foods to keep on a diet.

Children half-asleep in the morning may have a hard time getting down a large breakfast before school. Children need to eat more than two meals a day.

In addition to eating two meals a day, one should exercise on a regular schedule. The best combination of exercises is some kind of weight bearing exercise and aerobic exercise (Aerobic exercise gets your heart and breathing rate up for around thirty minutes and longer). When people do not exercise and go on a diet, they lose both muscle and fat! You need enough nutrition to support a program of exercise for losing fat and gaining muscle. To restrict calories without including exercise is likely doomed to failure. It is better to have positive lifestyle changes with purposeful exercise. This means having a positive exercise program that you enjoy daily.

Such as walking with friends, training for an event, or taking care of the yard and garden.

Currently, I enjoy lifting weights, and rock climbing, with hill walking as my exercise program. However, I am always changing my program for variety. For instance, I sometimes use an exercise bike or treadmill at home. What you do depends on your interests and hobbies. I find it better to have a hobby that depends on being in shape or incorporates healthy exercise when doing it. A good example is some form of martial arts training. I myself plan excursions to go mountain hiking or rock climbing during the weekends, so I train for this. I belong to a search and rescue group as a volunteer and this is my motivation to be in good physical condition. There are volunteer firefighter and search and rescue groups all across the world.

Find yourself an enjoyable physical hobby to train for, make it part of a positive lifestyle change. The new hobby will give you motivation to get in shape, lose weight, and keep it up. If you are unhealthy, a sudden extreme diet and exercise program could be harmful. See a health care provider, and read every book on the subject of health and exercise that you can find.

If you decide that two meals a day will not work for you, then you must think about counting calories. *For most people three full meals a day is too much food, then if you add in snacking then you are really over doing it.* There are many multiple meals a day diet programs and each need to count calories in some fashion, I personally find this is too much trouble. Nevertheless, find what works best for you.

A possibility while dieting is large midday snacking with very low glycemic index foods such as raw fruits and vegetables, with these you do not have to be as restrictive against snacking. However, you must avoid the high calorie health foods such as nuts, seeds and dried fruits midday when dieting. The advantage of this method is that it allows a large portion of complex carbohydrates into the system to satisfy nutrition and hunger. The need for this alternative depends on the individual. It may be helpful for those with an unstable eating schedule.

A lax two meals a day health plan that can work for some people with normal weight is two meals a day with unlimited mid day snacking: by *eating only* raw fruits, raw vegetables, raw seeds, raw nuts and healthy made olives. This variation does not let the organs rest in-between the main two meals, but it does fill the belly and allow healthy snacking mid-day. The digestion system can rest overnight between the evening meal and the breakfast meal. If you do this variation and have enough activity, it should keep weight stable, but you will not lose weight. This variation may work for people who do nervous snacking, which is eating because of stress.

If you find that you cheat some days on your program, it is not the end of the world. A treat on occasion will not kill a health program. Just get back on track the next day. Such cheating will not kill your diet unless it is too often. You may need a time of transition to get the two meals a day program to stick.

Remember, it is most important not to eat after the evening meal. If you are a little hungry at bedtime and at breakfast you are doing it right. The two meals a day diet program is best for adults after the age of twenty or so, depending on activity and physical condition of the person. Use some common sense. An overweight older teenager possibly can do this program but a lean growing teenager will need to eat more at mid-day.

Everyday visualize the kind of body you want to have and the activities that you want to do. The appearance you wish to have. This daily visualizing is part of the process of transition.

If you concentrate on eating pulse foods in a natural fresh condition, it will be easier to lose weight and keep it off for a lifetime. That means avoiding breads, meat, cakes, cookies, dairy products and most processed food products. Pay particular attention to avoiding manmade high glycemic index foods. Once you get the weight off you can experiment with adding back the non-pulse foods.

Homework, look up and list all the pulse foods you can eat while on your diet and also list the foods that are unhealthy, especially those you like. Post these on the refrigerator, load up on the good foods, and keep the bad foods out of the house.

Chapter Nine

The three pillars of better health

1. Diet
2. Exercise
3. Positive Mental State and Happiness

On the road toward better health, eating habits are just one part. The other main considerations are exercise and mental well-being. This is a triad of health where each leg is equally important as the other two. For health, you should eat well, have regular exercise and live well in a happy environment. For all of our lives we always can improve and change up hobbies and exercise programs to make life better and more interesting.

The three pillars of health.

One, have a clean diet with good nutrition.

Two, exercise, having a mixture of aerobic and anaerobic exercises. These are tied into fun active hobbies.

Three, happiness, this means to have a purpose and goals in life, being a positive person, living in a low stress environment. Happiness is mostly a daily positive habit.

All three pillars are equally important for health. The third pillar means being around positive people, living a positive lifestyle, having a moral code that is positive. No matter your economic circumstances, happiness is mostly up to your outlook, in having a life that has positive meaning.

Extreme stress may harm health as much as anything else, unhappy stress while eating can cause indigestion of food. Over a long time, this will destroy health and may cause ulcers even stomach cancer. I believe if you get the basic needs in life, such as a warm place to sleep, food to eat and a low stress lifestyle, then happiness is mostly a mental outlook problem. Even if exercise and diet are perfect, extreme stress will destroy health, an example is someone living with an abusive family member.

In western culture, we always seem to want more of something, to consume something, to win at something, to beat out others somehow, to be rich, famous and powerful. It is best to let these ideas go and enjoy what you do have, and concentrate on what you actually can achieve. For instance, I often get the shopping bug and I cruse the thrift stores and buy a few things and have great time while inexpensively consuming. I give unused items back to those thrift stores. This is how I can consume at times without busting the family budget.

I try to not to be caught up so much in politics, or religion in a negative way or trying to beat out others competitively. I try to avoid the win-lose mentality. Thinking I am happy only if I win and someone else loses. I try to have a win-win mentality where I can win and so can someone else and we both are happy.

If a person is chronically depressed, sometimes there is a physical problem, maybe an ongoing adverse reaction to something, or a lack of minerals or vitamins of some kind, maybe parasites, or something else physically wrong. Of course, an emotionally traumatic event in life causes normal unhappiness and depression for a time. Nevertheless, normal people work themselves out of this condition.

An extremely bad home life or work life or extreme poverty, can cause unhappiness. This is normal. Do the best you can to work yourself out of a negative situation. Unless they have chronic mental illness, most people are able to be happy. If you are chronically unhappy, look for causes, which have a real final cure. See a naturopath or an ecological doctor. I know that a lack of magnesium or ongoing allergic reactions to foods can cause depression and other mental problems.

Sometimes it is a copout by medical professionals to define a bad health condition as a mental health problem, when a physical cause is not easily found. Often a disease is named that is well known and there are drugs to forever treat it, but no one knows the real cause or has a real cure. In these cases, I suggest diligently researching in alternative medicine to try to gain better understanding of what is going on. I suggest never giving up, and keep on looking for a physical cause for illness and finding a real cure, ask God for help, and he will. Be patient.

To work toward a happier life also takes a method of transition. Each person and situation has different criteria. However, the general method of transition is the same, for instance if you are unhappy at work, look for better work. If you are unhappy at home, strive to find a better home life. Find friends that are more positive. Form a plan of transition, a method to make steady improvements. First study your own situation, and read all information sources that may be helpful. Then make a plan to work toward a better situation.

Try to find a purpose in life not tied up with greed or getting ahead of others. Try to stop the negative mental and physical repeating patterns that make you unhappy or angry. For instance, stop the negative mental loops that can fill your day, like getting mad every day at other drivers or mad at the other political side and so on. Change your daily negative mental habits toward something positive.

Being positive is a daily habit. Give thanks every day for something you do have and smile at someone every day. Give a compliment to someone every day. Say something kind to someone every day. Tell a funny story that is positive every day and so on.

The Biblical story of Namaan

Namaan was a great wealthy man who lived in Biblical times, he was the victor of many battles and was the highest general of the king in Syria. He was a handsome man and immensely admired and respected in his kingdom. Then, he became afflicted with the beginning stages of leprosy. In those days, it was a fearful disease with no cure. People who severely had this disease must dress in black to separate themselves from everyone else and often begged to survive.

In Biblical days, a victor of battle may take slaves and in Namaan's household, there was a slave girl who knew of a great prophet in her homeland. She, upon hearing the wife of Namaan crying about Namaan's leprosy told her about the prophet Elisha who may cure him. From this information, Namaan became hopeful and asked his king for permission to go for help. After receiving permission, he traveled to the king of Israel. Namaan thought he should go first to the King of Israel rather than the prophet because of the political power he had from his own king. However, he did not know this meant nothing to God. In fear, the king of Israel tore his clothes with terror because he did not know how to heal leprosy and did not think of Elisha. The king of Israel was fearful of the power of the king of Syria, and he could not cure leprosy. Therefore, Namaan's wealth and power was worthless in gaining a cure from God. This was a lesson for Namaan.

Elisha upon hearing about Namaan told his king to send Namaan to him and he will cure him through God. Therefore, Namaan traveled to Elisha and came to his household with a rich caravan with chariots and horses carrying gold, silver and spices. To receive this grand procession was a single disciple of Elisha, not Elisha himself! Standing outside in the doorway the disciple told Namaan to dip himself seven times in the river Jordan. That was it, nothing else! In those days, the river Jordan was a muddy river used by many people. Therefore, Namaan was greatly offended by the whole affair with this supposed prophet Elisha. He thought, "That man would not even receive me!" Nor would Elisha allow any gifts be given to him from Namaan, because he was only a messenger of God and Elisha knew it is God's blessing that heals.

Namaan went away very angry because of this affront to his position and intelligence. How could dipping seven times in the dirty river Jordon be a cure? Naaman was a proud man. He was proud of his accomplishments, talents, power, position, and wealth. It is ridiculous for him to think of it. The whole affair hurt his pride.

Nevertheless, the men and servants around Namaan talked to Namaan. They argued if Elisha had said to do some great task, would he not do so. He should try this cure, because there is no harm that will come from it.

Therefore, Namaan with nothing to lose and now understanding the test to his pride went to the river Jordan and dipped himself seven times and his leprosy instantly faded away. He was very grateful for a cure he cannot buy with wealth, power and position. The test he faced was the greatest kind that he personally could have confronted. A healing he could achieve only by humbling himself as directed by God. Afterward he lived a greater life, carrying a large amount of good in his heart to the world.

The second pillar-exercise, how to start

See your health care provider to consult about an exercise program.

If you are past the age of thirty, most likely exercise levels are too low. First, we need a shift in mindset, the typical person exercises to be stronger, faster and to win a contest. Many people exercise in order to beat others in competitive sports. In contrast, for health exercise is part of personal growth.

With this in mind, you need to start looking for positive hobbies that are exercise related. There are three categories of activities. First: those that are fun in themselves, second: to train for an event, or lastly a combination of the two.

One example is jogging in order to train for a race, or just jogging for enjoyment. It is best to have at least one hobby that requires you to be in good physical condition, this will inspire you to keep it up. Such hobbies are weekend mountain hiking, biking, backpacking, or community sports such as basketball, baseball, and tennis.

The exercise program should include full body muscle building as well as non-jarring aerobic or anaerobic body movements such as hill walking. Ideally, one should participate in an exercise activity several times a week for thirty minutes to an hour.

As an example, I will discuss my current hobbies and exercises. My main motivational hobby is mountain hiking and climbing. I hike, climb, or bicycle most weekends, one or two day trips. I also belong to a search and rescue group. This gives me extra motivation to be in physical shape.

During the week I play basketball, swim, and hike, ride an exercise bicycle, rock climb in the gym and lift weights, I like to change what I am doing week to week, and year to year. I like variety and to try new things in what I physically do. For instance I may rock climb less this year than the year before, but I will be doing more of something else like mountain hiking. For health, choose varying hobbies that are de-stressing and fun for you.

There are hobbies that you can choose that are sedentary and stressful. I suggest for health that you find active distressing hobbies. Any hobby that has you sitting and not moving very much is not conducive to one's physical health. For motivation to be in shape, consider joining a ski patrol or a local group that regularly exercises, for instance the boy scouts.

The mountaineers have a low cost program to train new climbers. Many climbing clubs have similar programs. In addition, think about training for a 10k run or a half marathon or an iron man race. Less dynamic goals could be training for seasonal mushroom hunting trips, sea kayaking, hiking trips or gathering medicinal plants. You can golf to be in shape, by walking the 18 holes, or join a martial arts class. I believe that without a related hobby most people will drop an exercise program in time.

One way to encourage exercise is to have a big goal. It can be a trekking trip abroad coming up in a year, or trying to climb a local mountain. Alternatively, to obtain a black belt in martial arts, there are plenty of martial art schools in most locations. There are also orienteering events in most areas that are conductive to be in shape, to exercise mind and body while navigating the course.

Another goal could be hiking sections of the Pacific North West Trail or the Appalachian Trail. An activity for older people or the partially disabled is to study Tai Chi, a Chinese martial art that is mild and therapeutic. It is fun exercise and one can try to become a Tai Chi master. Tai Chi is the gentle person's martial art. You could train in yoga; there are yoga classes most everywhere.

Ideas for healthy exercise are endless if you look for them. I have a push lawn mower and a large yard that needs mowing at least once a week in the summer. I often mow the neighbor's yard; this keeps me moving even when I do not feel like it. You can have a wood burning stove and gather the wood yourself.

If you are totally out of shape and do not know where to begin, start with walking and swimming. Walking is easier on the joints than running. Methods to increase the value of your walking are speed walking and hill walking. Since I mountain climb I like to walk stair steps or steep hills for exercise, sometimes with a light backpack. I get in a good workout without pounding my joints.

I picked up some exercise machines. A stationary bike, treadmill and elliptical machine, most of them I obtained cheaply second hand. I have them in front of the TV, and use them while watching. I exercise thirty minutes to an hour Monday through Thursday at night during the week. I strongly recommend trying this method; it is an especially good way to exercise in the winter months. It maximizes the time you have to exercise when it gets dark early evenings. These machines are easy on the joints. During the summer months, you can do walking, jogging, yard work and other outside exercises to change things up.

It can help to find an exercise partner or group in order to enjoy workouts. Most activities are more enjoyable with friends. Examples are many, martial arts, aerobics, stretching, walking, basketball, swimming, tennis, biking, yoga, and dance.

When starting out from scratch, first identify the hobbies and exercises that you would enjoy, try to identify light aerobic and full body muscle strengthening exercises. Keep in mind we exercise for health, although it is more enjoyable and fun if you have a related hobby or goal as well. You can write down possible goals on a list, and then start dreaming. Visualize becoming a black belt in martial arts or completing a mountain climb or finishing a 10k race, whatever. The best hobby is something that excites and challenges you.

Once you find your exercise related goal then work toward achieving it. The most beneficial hobbies are those that have a long-term goal, as well as short-term achievements. Examples are, mountain-hiking trips, mountain biking trips, backpacking trips, martial arts, ocean diving trips, golf without a cart, running foot races, yoga, caving trips and iron man races. If you find a physical hobby not working out for you or boring then change your program.

I personally like lifting weights, I have lifted weights at home in the past, but I have found that I do better if I have a separate location. I also like to rock climb indoors in the gym. The YMCA has good deals to join their gym and this is where I currently go. One can join exercise classes at most gyms and swimming pools with a structured schedule to follow.

I hung up a portable chin up bar in a doorway in my home. I do chin-ups most every time I walk through! You can find chin up bars in department stores or in the internet.

There are positive mentally active hobbies that are good for the mind, like playing chess, or reading and writing, but these are not physical for exercise. Balance out sedentary hobbies with physically active hobbies.

If you are a construction worker doing hard work you may want to rest during your time off-this is understandable. However, I know of a bricklayer whose hobby is the martial art Taekwondo. This works for him. Depending on the individual, find suitable hobbies and exercise levels.

An example of a non-suitable physical hobby is highway motorcycle riding; this requires skill and some endurance, but not so much in beneficial exercise. It is not a bad hobby in itself, but would need other hobbies for healthy exercise.

More on the third pillar, are you living a low stress happy life?

Are you happy? Are you a positive person? Are you fun to be around, do you have more positive thoughts than negative thoughts? Do you arrange your life around doing things (good) or buying things (bad)? Do you have positive friends or negative friends? Do you have a positive spouse? Do you enjoy your work? Do you have positive goals for the future? Are you a stuck in a rut? Are you self aware, can you change yourself to be a better person? If you answer any of these in a negative fashion, it will hurt health. All three legs of health are important. You are only as healthy as the weakest link.

After a certain age, most people stop growing internally as a person. Whatever they are out of high school or college, they seem to be stuck there for the rest of their lives. Most would rather cut off an arm than change their diet and lifestyle! To change lifestyle is a lot like changing your diet, it is best to work on it one-step at a time.

Let us begin with an important question: Are you happy, think about this a little. If you answered yes, and then go on. Many will answer no, if so let us analyze why. First you need to know what is making you un-happy, is it an illness, a stressful job, maybe poor family life? Only you know the answer. If it is something within your capacity to change, then the task will be much easier, in all cases, we must deal with our mental outlook. Ask God for help and pray, be patient and when an impression or something positive happens, be open to it.

There are many adverse events in life, which have the potential to ruin a day and longer. Mentally prepare yourself for these rough times so when they happen, it will not set a sour note. A tough boss may not go away, deal with it as positively as you can. Pay is for work, not for appreciation. Try to find better work and deal with what you have today.

The liberals will not change, neither the right-wingers, nor the bad people in your life. I find it best to go out of my way to have a light positive polite relationship with immediate neighbors, but not be excessively friendly. This approach works in the long term and will not risk sour relations forming up. Unfortunately, some neighbors are nasty or may become nasty quickly. The best method is to be polite and friendly to neighbors, but not try to become close friends too quickly, unless you want to take a risk.

In life deal with whatever you have today the best you can and try to change the situation for the better. I find that one should limit negative thoughts and activities, which are bad habits. If you become wound up like a rubber band when watching the news, then limit it. I rarely watch the news, and work on positive activities instead. If every day you are mad at slow traffic while driving, listen to classical music or to an educational book. Set your mind to avoid an endless unhappy habit, find ways to be more positive. Like all other positive lifestyle changes, this can be done step by step.

Walking, artistic painting or playing a musical instrument is great for relaxation. Volunteer at a local thrift store, food bank, church, school, boy scouts and fire department to find positive social interaction. Each person is different, find what works for you to be in a positive life.

Woodworking is relaxing and fun for some people, a small home repair project may be fun, or house painting or woodwork. If you do not know how to do something like automotive repair or home repair, get a few books to study about it. One hobby that could be fun and relaxing is restoring an old car or motorcycle. It is enjoyable to build models, maybe leading toward flying a model airplane, or running an electric model car.

Cheap relaxing hobbies are bird watching, fishing, geocaching, looking for wild plants and mushrooms, or walking a stream while fly fishing. Sewing is a great hobby, so is making jewelry. Change up hobbies when you become bored.

A pet is relaxing, but is a long-term commitment and may turn stressful later on. I notice many people choose hound dogs as pets. Be careful as hound dogs tend to run away from home and bark a lot. Many dogs bark a lot. Dogs need room to run, a fenced in yard is suitable. Having a pet is similar to having a child. You may have to find a babysitter for trips. I have two cats. Cats are better for me because they are independent pets.

Avoid non-relaxing hobbies. I would avoid gambling, smoking, coffee, drugs and alcohol. I avoid any activity where negative people are participating. I would not go into bars or nightclubs. What you get out of such activities are more than offset by bad experiences. Politics and religion can be negative hobbies, very often they are.

Are you a positive person? In life, it is very easy to get into a rut. Maybe you are self-programmed to be mentally negative, if so think how to break out of the negative thought pattern. The first step is to become self aware about what your thinking, saying and doing. Be honest, which may involve asking a friend to let you know when you are being negative. Often being negative is an automatic mental response to something that repeats endlessly. If so, work on reprogramming yourself to be more positive, even if it *kills you*. Then you will notice interactions with other people will be better. Not necessarily great, but better, smile when someone says hello to you, and say hello back.

If you are a negative person, try changing your behavior. If you pay close attention to yourself for a day, you may find that a negative thought pattern is an ingrained mental habit. A bad response that keeps repeating endlessly, like a virus in a computer program, stop it and change to a better mental habit. It will take time to change, but you can do it.

There have always been unfair situations in the world and always will be. How you live your life is still up to you. In other words, try to be ray of sunshine rather than a dark cloud. It will make the world a better place. More so than if, you try to influence people around you in a negative way, no matter your intentions.

Try to make it a habit to be positive. Suggestion: if you have an interest in news, politics, and find yourself being too negative because of it, then stop watching so much news and loose interest in politics, *at least in daily conversational life.*

If you have an un-healthy diet, or allergies or taking drugs of any kind, these will affect mood. If you are around negative stressful people and in negative employment, these will affect mood and health. Stress releases harmful hormones and prevents the digestion organs from functioning properly. If this happens daily, it will erode health. Even if you have diet and exercise perfect, too much stress will destroy your health.

Stressful people can be hard to deal with especially if they are in a controlling situation, like a senior family member or a boss in the work place. The first step is to try to control your mental response to those people, whatever it takes to reduce a stress reaction. The next step is to realize most people are not going to change. The stressful people around you are unlikely to be better in the future. Sadly, most people do not internally grow after their teenager years.

The most important step forward is to take more control over the bad situation. Work toward finding a way to restrict time around the negative person at work or home. For instance if you have a demanding older brother that you're working with in a job and it is making you sick, find another job and limit time with that brother. One of the toughest situations is when stuck with a demanding controlling person, such as an overbearing spouse.

A transition plan toward better life is working toward gaining confidence and becoming financially and emotionally independent. To stay in a bad relationship forever is a choice a person does not have to make. Try to make the relationship better and if this is impossible, can you live with it? If not, you must work yourself out of the relationship toward a situation where you have control over your life.

If the stressful relationship is with a relative, then often the practical solution is to limit contact to a single day a week, or even one day a month. From these ideas, you can find a solution. I would not cut off all relations to family because this is too severe. In most cases, it is best to keep family ties, but gain control over the situation. Find professional help and read every resource on this subject you can find.

Become aware of all outside and inside negative influences, and try to change as much as you can, try to deal with them in a better way. If you do this, you are on the transitional path to become a happier person. I am lucky to have a great spouse and a current job that is not so stressful. However, I sometimes become wound up over politics and news. I find it best if I do not watch the news; consider this yourself if you need to be happier.

If you are around negative people that are stressful to you, find a way to limit this contact. If your job is killing you, try to deal with it in a positive way and think about how to transition toward a better workplace.

Are you fun to be around? First let us identify the word fun. Do you make others happy, are you calming to be around? On the other hand, are you a know it all, an annoying bossy person? Can you listen as well as converse with people or must you do all the talking and bossing? Are you active or sedentary? Do you enjoy doing activities that positive people enjoy doing, or only what pleases you? Of course, it is easier to be a fun person when you are around people with similar interests. Nevertheless, it is better if we try to be compatible in new situations that are a little out of our comfort zone.

Do you have positive goals for the future? People without positive goals tend to be listless and aimless in life. This could easily lead to negativity and an un-healthy lifestyle. A positive person should have goals in life. What goals you have is a personal choice. A healthy dynamic person is always striving to learn new things and engaging in new fun activities or work.

Often older people loose interest in learning new things. Once you have lost interest in everything, you are in a downward spiral into old age. Remember to keep goals obtainable and work toward reaching them on a timetable. Do not create goals so far off into the future and so difficult that reaching them never happens. Try to choose goals that are fun, challenging and rewarding. For instance, an older person can learn to paint a landscape. That is a rewarding activity. Think of something fun to do *right now* that you have never done before. Find something out of your comfort zone; get out of your mental rut.

Examples: A fun goal might be learning to snowshoe; another rewarding goal might be learning a new language for a trip. Working toward a goal exercises the willpower muscle. As you strengthen willpower, this will enable you to reach other goals. If you feel you have no willpower, start small and stick to it.

Examples of simple lifestyle goals: give up a morning coffee for a morning herbal tea. Give up a morning of watching stressful news for a brisk walk with a friend. Instead of watching morning news TV, cook a tasty homemade lunch so you will not buy junk food.

In the evening while watching TV, why not exercise thirty minutes on a machine, no excuse except laziness. There are many exercise video programs to try as well. Alternatively, try thirty minutes of outdoor walking, or thirty minutes of any type of exercise. In general, for workout sessions thirty minutes of exercise is good, and go as long as an hour.

I do morning exercises during the week. They are a set of four exercises, usually push-ups, stomach crunches with other motions and stretching.

A common complaint is "I hate my job". Well, what are you doing about it? Sorry, playing the lottery does not count; God is not likely to reward you with a jackpot. Winning the lottery is up to chance and everyone's chances are the same-very low. Instead, think about what you can do to obtain employment that you like, maybe more schooling or starting a part time business.

Learn a new hobby in relation to health. For instance, build and use a small greenhouse, learn a new craft, such as cabinet building or boat building. The sky is the limit. At this point stop and think of one new hobby you would like to start this week.

Develop habits to create daily happiness. For instance, give thanks every day for something specific that you enjoy or appreciate. In Christian households, thanks are given at mealtime, at bedtime and several times during the day. This habit actually increases daily happiness. Every day try to smile three extra times. Make it a daily habit to do something fun and physically active for at least fifteen minutes. Each day try to reduce a negative influence.

Treat family, spouse, and good friends in a kind positive way, *all the time*, this will keep a social network. Going to the right church or social club is a way to build a positive social network. Happiness is not from money, or things, and getting over others. It is from a happy daily lifestyle. Happiness is a habit you live every day, only you can make that happen. There are many books and courses on the happiness subject, you can study and learn more.

Some cautions about a spiritual search, all religious organizations that strongly say, "We have a special privilege to God" are suspicious. Any religion or group that has special secret information or other secrets is suspicious. Any religion that is excessively money hungry is suspicious. Sometimes people are tied up into church politics and this becomes stressful, avoid this for yourself. I myself avoid church politics to keep a happy lifestyle.

Most con games entice people by *greed,* secret knowledge, position, and power for the mark. If a person, (con man) shows serious bad character to you just one time, most likely, they are going to cause you a lot of grief. Therefore, one time is enough in most cases to know to get away, unless you want to risk suffering.

Homework on lifestyle: Find resources to study a foreign culture you know little to nothing about, note the differences in lifestyle. Study about a different lifestyle that may be interesting, for instance mountain living in Alaska or the Himalaya. Find and read a biography that notes positive change in a real person's life. Like someone's transformation out of crime and prison toward something better.

In your hometown area, find at least three different kinds of lifestyles. For instance, city living to country living, differences in dress and activities between people of different ages and cultures. Recognize where you are at in terms of lifestyle and mindset as compared to other people. A very powerful education about lifestyle is emersion inside a foreign culture. An example is a city kid on a farm, or a country kid in the city.

Choose close friends carefully, not because they live next-door or happen to be in the circle of people you know. When you meet someone be friendly and polite. Judge their character and decide the kind of relationship you want with this person. For most people it will be polite and friendly, but not that close, set you mind for this. This is for people that you do not want to be that close to, because many people have poor character or are not compatible. Always judge character before deciding to try to become close friends. If you have a method of thinking through human relations, you will likely avoid bad situations

One may have a set of criteria to use when considering a new person to be close to in life. It is best to do some thinking before you try to be friends with someone, or risk suffering for it. For instance, find out if the person is honest. Find out if the person has the same general outlook in life, if they are somewhat the same in religion and politics. Find out if they like children and animals. Find out if they get along with their family, neighbors and current and past associates in work. Do they get along with other people in general? Find out their general disposition; is it neutral, upbeat or nasty? If you answer negatively to any of these questions, they are warning signs.

Some undesirable people will hide their true nature, but their past will tell the truth. Usually a person with a serious bad flaw in character has many others, all of which will make you suffer. When dealing with people you are around for the moment, but do not want to be close friends, it is best to be polite and friendly, but keep social distance. If you are the kind of person others should avoid, then work on your character. By the way, in judging others, we are not to judge them as if we are God. Our human judging is just for guiding our own lives. We do not have to suffer because of being around undesirable people. *However, only God can judge souls.*

Here are some personality types to avoid when making friends or romantic partners. Most everyone has bad personality traits to some extent. However, when extreme, bad traits can lead to suffering for you. If you ignore serious warning signs and still become close to someone, it will cause you pain. They say there is someone for everyone in romantic relationships, but I am not so sure. Do not be with someone in romance who will cause you suffering. Some people will have more than one bad personality trait. If you are a masochistic person (one who craves pain) here below is the list for you.

Narcissistic people: The world revolves around him or her. Can be difficult to recognize, as they may be flattering to get what they want. Nevertheless, in their mind the world rotates around them. To be friends with such a person will leave you used and abused. This type is hard to treat by psychologists.

Sociopathic people: Cunning and manipulative, they lack true emotion, but will act out emotions for what they want. They are often pathological liars and may lie every day of their lives. They see people as victims or accomplices for victims and don't have real in depth feelings of shame, remorse or guilt. Criminal behavior is possible and they may change their background or life story as needed. They often have promiscuous sexual behavior and may be child abusers. This kind of person leaves behind a broad wake of social destruction in their life, avoid or greatly suffer. Beware, they are very skilled in hiding their true nature.   (Maybe most politicians are sociopathic?)

Extremely emotional people: These people need love and attention far greater than normal. They are over emotional and may react out of proportion to some social situations. As friends or lovers, they can be exhausting by being too needy and unstable (clingy, crying, flirting, mood swings, etc). They tend to have depression mixed in with over emotionality. Psychologists can treat this personality type to some extent.

Passive-aggressive people: They are hot then cold toward others, will entice, then withdrawal when they get a response. They are big on the silent treatment as punishment. They give double messages, come closer and move away. To play with such a person will have you manipulated and off balance all the time. They may run late to appointments to make others wait. The usual cause of this behavior is unexpressed anger. They are very adept in hiding their true nature.

Obsessive-compulsive people: They may excessively worry about whether if they turned out the lights or not when leaving home. They may throw a fit if something is out of place on their desk or at home or somewhere else. They may have chronic self-doubt and endlessly check certain things. They may be neat freaks, and or endlessly repeat words and ideas while speaking or writing. May be serially obsessive, and become hooked on an idea or project and totally focus on it. They must finish it before they can move on. This type of person may be driven by the need for control. In relationships, they may be distant and remote in order to control their emotions. They may have or develop an alcohol or drug addiction, or eating disorders.

Mood-swing people: They run hot then cold in their moods. They may cling to friends, and later on angrily push them away. May tend to use people and have an addictive personality toward drugs, alcohol, smoking, coffee, food and gambling. May be accident-prone, and unable to spend an evening home alone. A relationship with such a person will mean a rough up and down ride. This condition is serious if manic then depressive. It may be related to diet deficiencies, such as a lack of magnesium, or chemical imbalances. This person can try to eat a balanced diet, and take supplements to get into chemical balance. It is best to get professional help.

Depressed people: It is normal to be down for a while when life becomes rough. However, when depression is chronic it is time to be concerned. Depressed people can bring everyone down around them and may be needy. Depression may be linked to chemical imbalances, which may be helped by better diet and or supplements. Severe depression is serious and needs professional help. A warning sign for you is meeting someone who is taking anti-depression medications. If they go off the medication personality changes may happen, often from bad to worse. Medications have side effects so many depressed people do not want to take them long term. Some people on medication may get even more unstable. Suicide is possible especially for the chronically depressed.

Paranoid and or insecure people: This type of person tends to be suspicious of everyone and everything. They think someone is out to get them or romantic partners are cheating on them. They are unable to trust people and feel insecure all the time. They will be suspicious of friends and romantic partners, thinking they are cheating or sneaking around behind their back.

Addictive people: Addiction can come in many forms; the most serious kinds are to alcohol and drugs. Sadly, most people are set in their ways after their teenager years. It is not possible to save an addict from the outside. Addicts must want to change themselves and do most of the heavy lifting to achieve sobriety. Such a person is on a rough roller coaster ride in life. Do not hop on with them unless it is true love...

Just plain idiot people: We all run into these types from time to time. They never get their life in order and a wake of social destruction follows them around. They may seem fine on one level, but are often very needy. They are endlessly bumbling along in life, from one disaster to another. Do not get caught up in their lives. Do good deeds to help them out if you desire, but hang around too long and you will suffer. Often they will cling like glue to anyone who is a life raft.

Abusive people: They are manipulative, may lie and fake kindness and interest in you to get into a domineering abusive relationship. They can be verbally or physically abusive or both. They often have learned abusive behavior from parents or siblings and others. It is best not to start a serious relationship with someone with strong signs of abusive behavior. They often hide their true nature. Then when living with someone or married the real abuse begins.

This is a short list. You should do more research if you notice odd or extreme behavior from anyone. Remember, people often hide unfavorable behaviors. When starting a romantic relationship it is a good idea to identify the personality of the person. It may be helpful to know the personalities of the parents, grandparents and their extended family. Sometimes personality traits skip a generation.

I am mildly obsessive compulsive and my wife claims that I am a hypochondriac (health phobias). What are you?

Chapter Ten
Self awareness

Are you self-aware? Many people are not self aware, often those who need to be the most are not. To start being self-aware simply look in the mirror and ask, "Who am I"? Do you like yourself? If not, is it time to change?

A sad but common pattern of a non-self aware person is being annoying to others in a way that they cannot stand happening to themselves, like being a bossy pushy person. A non-self aware person does not understand why no one likes them, because they do not recognize their own negative behavior. If you want to become a more positive person, be more self aware when interacting with people.

How can a person become self-aware? First step is to understand yourself. Look at the list of bad personality traits given in the last chapter. If honest, most of us will see some of these in ourselves, hopefully not to an extreme degree. Learn to be aware of your own personality traits and work on improving them. If you want to be a positive person, I suggest, emulating positive self-aware people, and limiting influences from negative non self-aware people.

Self-aware people carefully choose their words and actions; non self-aware people talk endlessly, tend to blurt out words and actions. It is easier to be a positive person when around positive people. Be one of the positive people.

Any time you are interacting with someone and it is negative because of you, try to change your behavior to make it more positive. Sadly, negative people tend to be the least likely to try to change for the better. One can try to change them from the outside, but most people will not change unless they want to. Most people have their personality traits set at a young age and are unable to grow. Nevertheless, if a person wants to be happier they should study this subject and work to change.

In diet and lifestyle, it is important to be self aware of your own body, to understand cause and effect all the time. If you eat something that gives a negative reaction, then you should be able to tell it right away and mentally trace back to possible causes. Work on your mind-body, and food-body mental self-awareness. Also, pay attention to your loved ones, they may not have skills in this area. For instance, if your child develops a migraine after petting an animal, it may due to an adverse reaction to the animal.

An example of being self-aware: A stressful day at work tenses up your neck muscles, also breathing in chemical fumes causes a migraine. You should recognize such events when they happen. In daily life, you want to note and understand these instances and to treat and prevent them the best you can. When home you can take some activated charcoal and take a walk to unwind.

Strive to understand the food-body connection. Do certain foods make you feel bloated, constipated, and ill in any way? Most people have limited mind food-body self-awareness. They do not actively feel the connection when feeling good or bad with daily interactions with food and environment. Most people are passive about how good they feel, they only notice when feeling extremely bad. If you clean up your diet and environment, your food-body self-awareness will increase.

An example of being self aware, I notice that I have better mental function when I get plenty of vitamin B and lecithin. Paying attention to proper nutrition while eating good food will help a student in school. Lecithin is a healthy fat that will help the brain recover when studying.

If you are an athlete in training, can you feel your body and know when you need to rest or have more training? If your muscles are sore, can you tell if you need more protein, or extra rest, or both? If your muscles are cramping, do you know what your body needs? Do you need more salt or other minerals and in what combination and how much? In reality, it is difficult to tell these things by only feeling your body. You may need blood work and professional help. However, you can do much with mind-body self-awareness.

Another example is an allergen attack. If you feel a headache coming on and start throat clearing, stop and think, "What caused it"? Usually people just keep on working and ignore the onset of an allergen attack or illness. However, if you stop to think about the immediate past and pay close attention, often you can figure out the causing agent. Is it a pet allergy or an allergy caused by a certain food, or is it a chemical in something like a cosmetic, or from something else? Consider self-testing. Self-testing is adding and removing items from the diet and environment to see how you feel, better or worse. For example, if you suspect a certain item is making you feel bad; you remove it and see how you feel. Usually in time with self-testing, you can figure out the cause and eliminate the problem. If you do not make this effort, such adverse reactions may destroy health over time.

The most important single lesson to learn from this book is how to be more mind body self-aware. To know how to detect and remove those drinks, foods, pharmaceuticals, supplements, herbs, social situations or chemicals that are causing bad reactions and ill health.

To be more self aware in practice is very simple. Do you feel good at this moment? If yes, think about how you slept, ate and drank during the time beforehand. Think about the people you were around, what you were doing, everything. Remember all these things, to reflect and think about them.

Alternatively, do you feel bad right now? If yes, then think about what feels bad. For instance if you have a bellyache, think about what you ate. You may figure out the cause and prevent it from repeating. This is the goal.

Maybe you have a migraine. Is it because of something you ate, breathed in or had on your hands and rubbed onto your face?

Do you have a skin rash that will not go away? It could be due to a food allergy, maybe from eating too many nuts or berries. Itchy skin anywhere on the body is often due to an allergy from something put into the mouth.

Do you have a sinus headache? It could be an allergic reaction to a pet, or from breathing in diesel exhaust fumes or from something else.

Every type of ill feeling has a set of most likely causes to seek out and eliminate. Any health problem can be an adverse reaction to a food, beverage, and pill or something in the environment.

Mind body self-awareness means paying attention to how you feel all the time, good, bad, or neutral and understanding why. If you feel good in a certain environment, and when eating certain foods and getting enough sleep, remember this and try to continue into the future. Oppositely, if you feel bad, try to figure out why. Then experiment as needed to improve. For instance if I realize I have a headache and I am working around paint fumes, I may take three activated charcoal capsules and put on a respirator. Do not ignore bad health events because they will erode health over time.

In western culture, most think it proper to be tough, macho and ignore pain, toxins, loud noises and more. Remember these adverse events will reduce real strength and may destroy health in a short amount of time. For example, you can breathe in chemical fumes, and be tough for a moment, then weak, and sick for the rest of life. Be careful of making this kind of choice. Watch what you do in the workplace. Few jobs are worth a lifetime of sickness. Only you and your close family really care about you.

If you are tired, can you stop and let yourself rest, rather than push until illness and physical breakdown? Are you able to have an open mind if someone mentions a poor habit that you have? Are you willing to explore a positive lifestyle change? Often positive changes do not stick right away, but keep on trying by making small steps. Do not forget the mind-body connection, if you are on any type of drug, herb or supplement, it may affect your mood. Vitamin and mineral deficiencies can affect mood and mental health in a negative way. A possible cause of mental problems such as depression and bi polar is nutritional deficiency.

Lessons from my personal experience in mineral deficiency: I found that distilled water is not good for exclusive long term drinking. Distilled water if drunk for too long can leach out vitamins and minerals. Distilled water is pure H_2O, and spring/well water has minerals dissolved inside of it. Long ago when living with my brother for three years. I drank only distilled water because his well water tasted bad with high sulfur content. I eventually became anemic from lack of iron, magnesium and other minerals and had to go on supplements. Unfortunately, I was not able to tell this ill affect while it was happening, so there are limits to mind body self-awareness.

Most of the time mind body self-awareness will work to save you, but not every time. Only afterward, when I was anemic in iron I understood what happened. You cannot always depend on mind-body self-awareness to prevent permanent damage to your body from toxins or a bad diet practice.

Distilled water is good for short term cleansing, maybe for a few days up to a month. If you drink distilled water long term, you must add in extra supplements, full spectrum vitamins and minerals to replace what you lose by diuretic effect. Drinking distilled water is acceptable short-term, for instance in some cases of kidney illness because it is easier on the kidneys.

Another personal case: Years ago I drank too much caffeinated tea over a long time and this created painful crystals in my kidneys. Afterward, I found out in a health book that this happens often enough to people, depending on genetics. Therefore, a person may be eating or drinking something that they think healthy, but is not. Both cases, in drinking distilled water and drinking excess green tea. I thought I was doing something healthy and then learned afterward that I made a mistake.

These instances happened to me due to a lack of information in my *current health* resources I had at the time. This is why I think it is important to research widely using many information sources and always let how you feel be the final guide. Watch how you feel, for any slight adverse effect, to be noted quickly and corrective action taken.

When feeling ill your body cannot tell you directly why, so you must hunt down the reason. A procedure is to pray to God for help. Then study every resource you can on health and join internet discussion forums that seem appropriate. Try elimination programs from foods, drinks, supplements and environmental items. Eliminate all suspect items and bring them back in a testing way. Look for deficiencies in diet, for anything needed in the body, such as enzymes or healthy intestinal flora. Consider bacterial, viral or parasite causes of illness. Go to health care professionals for diagnosis, but do not be a helpless sheep, be proactive. Research all drugs for side effects and their time on market.

It is best to know if you are a test subject with new drugs on market. Be extra leery about any drug on the market less than ten years. You can find books and resources about drugs on the internet. Research all medical procedures; know the true success and failure rates. Know the percentages of false negatives and false positives for medical tests.

Chapter Eleven
What is moderation?
What is healthy?

Some people say they are on a health diet, but sometimes they are on a restrictive unhealthy diet. As you learn more about health and different kinds of diet programs, you will run into oddball health programs. I think we all are sincere in trying to be healthy. What lifestyle to live is a matter of personality, opinion and different information sources.

Every health expert has differences and these can be major. However, if you are getting enough protein, fat, balanced nutrition, vitamins, minerals, and carbohydrates in a healthy unprocessed digestible form, then you are on a healthy diet plan. I suggest reading widely and always consider that you are making a mistake if you are not feeling well.

If you are on a program that is far away from what most health experts are advising, you may want to reconsider and reflect on how you feel. In progression toward better health there are always new things to try and new variations to experiment with, for instance in recipes and supplements. How you feel should be the guide as you make these changes, while understanding that sometimes-adverse effects take a long time to be noticeable.

I am cautious of any manmade

supplementation, especially of anything new to me. I am cautious of any strong herbal treatment to be used long term. I am more open to gentle natural diet changes for health. These are less risky and usually all that is needed.

I know someone who had heart problems who decided because of prompting by the spouse that a low salt diet was the way to be heart healthy. Therefore, he went to extremely low salt intake and after a time had severe muscle cramping in the legs at night. He found this went away after taking salt tablets. So be very careful when making any kind of diet change. Adding things in or taking things away in excess may cause an adverse effect. This bad effect may slowly sneak up on you.

The human body is wonderful, but it cannot tell you directly what is right or wrong in diet and environment. You must figure it out from internal and external how you feel clues, by research and testing. It can take hours, days and even years to figure out what is going wrong in health. For instance, a vitamin deficiency can cause severe illness over time, and have a simple cure, but the body cannot tell you directly what is wrong.

A common mistake by people who are trying to be healthy is they overeat or under eat particular items in diet. One can have too much or too little of many things in diet such as proteins, salts, fats, sugars and carbohydrates and with many types of vitamins and minerals. If a person is on an oddball system and forces themselves to eat in an unbalanced way, this is unhealthy. Usually you can tell such a person, because they have a strange diet system and are unhealthy. If someone is unhealthy, be careful about following his or her diet advice. Usually you can tell this because they look unhealthy in some fashion.

In any case, there are many paths to be healthier, so be tolerant of other people. The more broadly you read, the more grounded you will be to judge. I have found every health expert to have areas of fantastic information, but all missed something.

I think the safest way to take vitamin supplements long term is by a pre-balanced formula. I like the whole food vitamins the best. Then the vitamins that are made from whole foods. Lastly, vitamins made chemically. My sensitive kidneys can only handle some kinds of whole food vitamins. Because they are not as concentrated and are the most gentle. For long-term health, as in decades of using supplementation, I suggest only whole food vitamins and minerals. These may save your organs from slowly being damaged. It may be even better to get nutrition only from food for the longest healthy life span. It takes extra effort to have a complete nutritious diet with only food, but I think this is the best way, just like Biblical Daniel. Manmade supplementation may unknowingly damage organs over a long period of time.

Good health takes extra effort by eating plenty of organic raw foods and lightly cooked foods. This means mostly raw fruits, raw vegetables, raw nuts and raw seeds with some cooked grains. This is why I suggest all snacking to be of natural foods, in the least processed form for nutrition.

Most people into health try out high doses of vitamins and supplements and herbs at times. Every single instance to date when I have tried this for myself, after a few weeks to months, I stopped the practice, and I felt better. On average, I think it best for me to take a health supplement, vitamin, or herb into the body for a while (if I need it), let us say for a month or less and then I end it.

For me, strong herbal treatments should be ended in about two weeks as a rule of thumb. If you are taking a single vitamin or mineral due to deficiency, most likely you will want to end it after a time. If someone is deficient in something, it may be good to go reasonably high with a supplement dosage, then afterward to use a balanced formula, if anything at all. Too much of any single mineral or vitamin may throw the body out of balance, just like being deficient of a single mineral or vitamin.

The same caution with some food items. We may hear from a health expert that a concentrated natural item is good for you. Alternatively, a health study says a certain vitamin is great for health. However, long-term effects are unknown in any short-term science study. I suggest being cautious when taking anything with strong effect such as vitamins or supplements especially with high dosages for a long time.

There are people chronically deficient due to poor diet and lifestyle choices. A drinker of coffee, tea, and soda may be chronically deficient in minerals due to the diuretic effect of their drinking habits. A person who will not change their harmful beverages may need to use supplementation at a slightly higher level in an on going basis. If so, it is best to find professional help and use the least harmful supplementation.

In all deficiency cases, it is best to create a better diet. Eat plenty of greens and vegetables daily. It is almost as powerful as juicing to boil greens for a short time (five minutes or so). They will reduce down in size. Then eat the greens and drink the water the greens are cooked in.

A personal supplementation example: I took Iodine for a few months-about two drops a day for health, lack of Iodine is a common deficiency. Nevertheless, I decided to limit this practice and I feel great, I cycle off and on the iodine supplementation. How to cycle off and on supplementation has no fixed rule. It depends on your body and nutritional needs. Remember, any nutrient in excess over time may go from a good effect to bad effect because of throwing the body out of balance.

It is tricky to work out supplementation cycles by only feeling your body by cause and effect. One could do blood tests if you can afford them. It is a good practice in general not to over do any single strong supplement. In other words anything much stronger than found in nature naturally. If taking something for a long period, there is a risk of overdoing it and not knowing until bad effects appear.

A rule of thumb is to use a balanced mild herbal, vitamin, mineral, or protein formula for long-term supplementation. Although if you have a bad reaction from one of the ingredients in the formula you cannot tell which one it is. I sometimes take a balanced whole food vitamin complex. However, a person can take no supplements at all and may have *better* health. For the last year, I have been taking only one supplement-vitamin D, and feel great. The danger of any supplement, even those made with the best ingredients and intentions is it may have something harsh in it due to processing.

If I had chronic health problems, and could not figure out why on my own I think conventional medical diagnosis is great to try. However, I try to avoid using drugs or harsh medical treatments to regain health. I am suspicious of any medical diagnosis that has no final cure. That is a cop out in my thinking. Other than a few rare instances, I believe diseases have a real cure-if you know what to do. Do not give up and do not trust any information source a hundred percent, keep learning and exploring. Ask God for help and listen for the answering impression.

Defining moderation

I put some thought into this question, what is a moderate consumption of anything, how to define it? If you define a moderate consumption of sugar by the average intake of sugar in the USA, then about 180 grams a day would be acceptable! However, if we consider there is an epidemic of diabetes in the USA and the ancient human consumption of sugar is somewhere around eight grams a day. Therefore, if you were going to define moderate consumption of sugar according to ancient man's consumption it would be about eight grams a day. Therefore, if you consume a single 12oz soda, it alone would have about five times as much as the moderate amount of ancient man's sugar consumption. With these numbers, it is easy to understand why the average amount of sugar eaten daily in modern society may destroy health.

So what is truly moderate in consumption for your body, verses what is considered moderate in the culture of today? Think on this.

It is not excessive to drink one soda a day, is it? However, one may think that the design of the average human body is only to handle eight grams of sugar a day, not 180 grams of sugar. So what is a moderate amount of sugar for good health opposed to what everyone is doing? We can see that what is acceptable in modern society, that your body may not recognize it as moderate!

If you carry on this line of reasoning, what else we consider moderate in modern society, which in reality is too much? Several cups of coffee a day is moderate-right? Eating a couple pastry products a day made from sugar and hardened fats is moderate, right? Maybe a milk chocolate bar every day, is this moderate as well? Some can consider a few drinks of an alcohol beverage every day to be moderate. In reality, is the body designed for a modern day *moderate* consumption of many items?

Clearly, there is no exact definition of moderation for us to follow. However, consider your own family genetic history and the exotic to you foods, those that are new to your genetic history. These kinds of exotic to you foods are more likely to cause problems and adverse reactions, especially in excess.

The ancient human diet, on average is made up of some clean lean meat, and tubers, fruits, seeds, and nuts along with some simple food products made from these, mostly baked or fermented foods. Later on in time people started to use coarse grains so we have some human history with these. Therefore, we may eat some of the least processed natural grain products. Some people think if you stray too far from your body's historical diet you will get into health trouble.

For example, *only one soda a day* may put you way over the ancient diet in terms of daily sugar consumption. Think about other common food or drink items, such as coffee, or out of area exotic to you vegetables, fruits and grains, also genetic modification, pesticides, hormones and food additives. Negative effects are possible from any exotic to you food or drink item. It can be an acute reaction or build up slowly over a long time. It is good to consider everything that you ingest on a regular basis in this light.

Some food or drink items of the non-ancient category may be harmful and others not so bad, it depends on individual genetics and how much ingested. However, on average, I would not eat a large amount of non-ancient for your body foods on a daily basis. Avoid or limit those items that are not in your personal historical family diet.

Your individual genetic history will determine much of what you can safely eat. Only in recent times foods and drinks are made and distributed all over the world. In addition, people have the ability to move to new locations of the world, where their body's genetics has no long-term history with local foods, drinks and pathogens. Even a generation or two in a new location in the world is not that long in terms of human genetics and family history.

They did not have coffee in the ancient days, or processed sugar products. Most people cannot digest cow's milk as adults; suggesting dairy is not in their family's historical diet. Chocolate, was not around in the ancient days for most people. Chocolate originated in South and Central America. Genetic engineering of food is very new; from one year to the next, it can change foods.

Many forms of processed grains and oils, like white wheat products and genetically altered oils were unknown for consumption even a few decades ago. An ingested item or two a day, which is socially acceptable, may harm your body.

Often we find out that we ingested too much of something harmful only after the fact. However, if you watch closely how you feel, you will notice an ill effect coming on and getting stronger, and then you can act to eliminate it.

If I eat a chocolate bar or drink a soda, I normally choose the healthiest versions and ingest them at most once a week. I think it is better to ingest these items less than once a week. How much to consume in foods and beverages is something you must decide for yourself. The most important thing is to be aware.

I am sometimes offered a soda in social situations. I do enjoy the taste of soda pop and the slight caffeine high off it. In such social situations, I try to limit it to one a day and try to pore half of it out when people are not looking. This is to be social, and to have a positive interaction with others. Ingesting such items a little on occasion is fine. Most people will be upset if you try to talk health to them at such times, and bluntly refuse the item. It is better to be a gentle positive health influence on other people.

I choose to be as healthy as I can, and to have very low tolerance for un-healthy items. I may have a piece of chocolate occasionally or single cup of coffee if I am driving at night and sleepy, or rarely have an ice cream cone. I am aware of what I am doing, so should you when making such choices.

An example of how bad the average diet can be, by what is considered moderate in modern society. From a 2005 US News and world Report the average USA citizen consumes 142 pounds of sugar a year. The primary sources of sugar are from beets, cane and corn. Before processed sugars, ancient peoples used to eat about eight grams of fructose sugar a day (according to Linus Pauling). Today the average sugar intake is up to 176 grams a day in the USA!

Sweeteners are just one of many items

added into processed foods that are not in the original Biblical diet. I consider it more harmful to eat a diet high in processed sugars, than a diet high in clean fresh meat, if I had to choose between the two extremes. Therefore, if you restrict meat intake and still eat processed sugars and carbohydrates, I do not consider this practice to improve health. Think about it, humans have an ancient history of eating meat in quantity at times, not with processed sugar and other processed products. Therefore, to eat vegetarian for health with no other consideration is not healthy. I know of people who think they are eating healthy by not consuming meat, but they are making mistakes elsewhere.

High sugar intake along with other processed grain and fat products promote diabetes, obesity and heart disease, more so than clean meat products.

The ancient history of the human race is a small daily intake of fructose sugar. Think about it, where would people obtain bulk concentrated sweet foods out of season in the old days? Clean saturated animal fat is not as dangerous for health as eating a lot of sugar. Some saturated fat is not harmful and I use a little organic butter at times. Of course, a diet high in meat is not ideal either. It is a matter of degrees.

Just last night as I am editing this section of the book, I ate some processed sherbet products and they tasted great. (Of course, I broke my not eating after the evening meal rule; we all are human...) Then I felt bad the rest of the evening until bedtime. I understand I have a bad reaction to this processed treat. My wife loves these so she will be disappointed, but I have to avoid them. Moderation for me in this context means none of these treats.

These days it seems that there is an epidemic of people in chronic sickness. Most humans cannot handle today's exotic sugars, and processed grains in the quantity they are consumed. I do consider beet sugar and corn syrup to be exotic foods because people don't have a long-term history eating these.

There are thousands of food additives and genetically modified processed foods in our food supply. There are traces of pesticides, hormones and antibiotics in many foods. If it is processed you are ingesting toxic food, our bodies are not designed to eat these kinds of foods.

I think we are going through a kind of genetic weeding out process in this modern age. Rapid changes in food are a problem for humans, if the rate of change is too great, can people adapt fast enough? Is this God's plan? I think not, his plan is natural food as close to the original form as possible. Slowly changing food is the safest way.

Example, my wife and I went to a party, they offered me a soda, fine I thought, I will have a 12oz soda. I shared this with my wife, and I ate some cake. Remember the ancient human diet had about eight grams a sugar a day. A single 12oz soda has 39 grams of sugar; (a 20oz soda has 65 grams of sugar). Therefore, that would be about 20 grams of sugar for both my wife and I, and we both ate some pastries. I would guess we both ate at least 30 grams of processed sugar.

That is about four times above an ancient daily consumption of sugar. We were being very limited in what we ate and we still ate excessive sugar as compared to an ancient diet. Now you can understand why there is an epidemic of obesity and diabetes and heart disease. There is a correlation with sugar intake and heart disease. Count your grams of processed sugar intake today, for most people it is way above eight grams.

A single 20oz soda will net you 65 grams sugar, then add in one pastry, let us say a single donut; we want to be moderate, right? A donut has 12 grams of sugar making 77 grams of sugar for our *moderate* snack. This could be called being restrictive in today's world.

Nevertheless, this amount of processed sugar alone is almost a 1000 percent over the ancient human consumption of eight grams of sugar a day! In short, most human bodies are unable to handle so much sugar daily and keep healthy. Furthermore, I suggest to not simply replace sugar with artificial sugar substitutes, as most of these are harmful in excess.

In this chapter, I assume that 8 grams is the amount of sugar our bodies are designed to ingest daily. It could be another number, even double or triple eight grams. Even so most people in modern society are still eating too much sugar and refined grains to be healthy.

Chapter Twelve

How to consider sources of information

When reading differing sources of information, what to believe? Sadly, there is scientific information and expert advice to support almost anything you wish to believe. If you want a King Nebuchadnezzar kind of diet and lifestyle, there will be sources that say that is fine. An example is coffee, some health sources say it is good and others say it is harmful, so you can choose what you wish to believe. I suggest always be gathering information and use common sense and be self-aware. Most often personality will decide for people what they believe to be healthy without much thought or experimentation. I use my own experience as the primary guide, for coffee. I find it is fine as a short-term stimulant. However, when I use it daily I have less overall energy and my mental function suffers.

In regarding scientific health studies, these are good information. However, be careful, often there is bias and short term positive results may not mean much for long-term health. Most health studies do not give a full picture of what is going on. You should think about all the information given. For instance, vitamin C is good for you, but too much vitamin C will leach calcium out of your body. This information is rarely given and is not on any vitamin C supplement bottle I have seen. Therefore, if you take high dosages of vitamin C long term you may need supplementation with calcium and make sure all other minerals are in balance.

In the past, even some doctors said smoking is healthy, so you have to be on your toes with any information about health. Every person has a different body type; people will react differently to foods and toxins. Every person has a different history of toxins inside their body. For instance, we all should eat fruits and vegetables, but a person with rheumatoid arthritis should restrict intake of the nightshade family of vegetables. What will work for one person and is healthy, may not work for another.

In health studies, you must consider the context of a study. High levels of a single vitamin or a supplement may help a study group during a short time frame. Nevertheless, such results may have no connection to long-term good health. A study or research may show a good effect, but the item may be unhealthy over a longer time. Usually a study has an unstated goal by those who are paying for the study. The study may be honest, but still have an angle they are trying to prove.

For example, there are two conflicting ideas regarding meat, one-meat is not good for you, and the other says meat is important for nutrition. Both sides have some truth in their thoughts and writings. I have seen healthy people who were vegetarians; for instance a sixty five year old Asian man who could run as if he was in his twenties. I also have seen unhealthy looking vegetarians. Alternatively, I have seen healthy meat eaters. I also have seen heavy meat eaters in horrible health condition.

Such a mixture of personal experiences can be confusing. One must consider the whole picture. Most people who eat little meat tend to be more health conscious than heavy meat eaters are. Is this noted in personal experience or in a study? Did the meat eaters eat a little clean meat in their diet and otherwise eating very well? We may try to compare them to a group of vegetarians eating no meat, but are eating many bad processed foods. You can see that unstated variables in a health study may have overwhelming importance. There are many possible differences in what people eat, so the meat verses no meat debate alone leaves out important variables in gauging diet and lifestyle.

A study may not show the full situation about a supplement which is being studied. Consider a study about taking high amounts of vitamin E, and the benefits or detriments of this practice. How long was the study? Are there any other variables in the study not mentioned?

When considering a supplement or diet and anecdotal (from personal experience) information and studies, try to see the big picture and consider short-term gain compared to long-term health. Consider organ health as important to have a long life span. An example is alcohol. This is a drug and toxin, short-term the body can handle it, but years of excess will destroy the liver. The same mistake can happen in a bad diet practice or when using supplements. You may tolerate it for years, but destroy long-term health.

Many say drinking red wine from grapes is healthy. However, the grape is the main source of benefit, not the alcohol.

Once you harm an organ, it may be difficult to get its health back to a hundred percent. Most often, you cannot, and it is the weak link in health and lifespan. You can live only as long as the weakest link allows you in terms of vital organ systems in the body.

I think in general, anything modified or man made with high heat processing is not as good as fresh or frozen. Most frozen foods are frozen when the fruits and vegetables are ripe at the time of freezing, which is good. Anything chemically made, even supplements are not as good as pure food for long-term health. The longest living healthiest people of the world do not take supplements. They eat a pure balanced diet and exercise in a low stress lifestyle. Anything that is processed is risky to consume long term. I prefer ingesting the least processed foods and beverages as much as possible. Modern genetic engineering is a real risk to health and may cause adverse reactions. Longer-term effects need extended experiments to know for sure. I personally do not want to be a live test subject, by being part of a weeding out process that is going on now. This is happening due to the altered food supply, along with human sloth, gluttony and carnal desire.

It is better to use natural foods and supplements as natural as possible. It is best to pace yourself in life and exercise, not to push to hard and cause an acceleration of your cellular death rate.

Vitamins are important to health, so are minerals. The best source for them is in foods and beverages, then from whole food supplements. The chemically made vitamins may be hard on your organs and prematurely age them. I am very cautious of artificial foods or supplements. A health study may say a supplement item is great during the period of the study, but still be cautious of long term usage-especially at high dosages.

My general thought on herbs and homeopathy treatments; I think these may be fine for acute treatments for disease or sickness. However, I would strive to heal myself long term by better diet and lifestyle as much as possible.

For longer-term health, I shy away from using strong herbal treatments in an on going basis. The exception to this rule is the milder herbs that are also foods. Garlic, onions, cayenne pepper, and other herb foods may be safely used long term. It is best to use food herbs to pleasant taste and not excessively, especially long term.

Let how your body feel be the ultimate guide and do careful research before taking strong herbs. The makers of herbs and supplements are not allowed by law to say what they are good for on their packages in some countries (USA). This means you need to seek out information to know what they are good for, proper dosages, side effects, how and when to cycle off and on. Seek out professional help and study information sources as needed.

For best health, focus on proper diet, food

selection, fresh air, exercise, sunlight, rest and good companionship. Herbs, homeopathy, and even chiropractic treatments all have their place in healing. However, I would not replace pharmaceuticals with herbs or homeopathy treatments and end my search for improving health.

Sometimes a person is addicted to an item that causes an allergic reaction. If you are in a bad health condition and notice that you are eating foods that are on an allergen-causing list, you may be sickly because of these and not know it. It can take a week or two (possibly even longer) of abstaining to clear out allergen foods and chemicals from you body, to get in a condition where you can tell if you are having an allergic reaction to something specific. In addition, you can have blood tests and other tests from a physician to test for allergies or adverse reactions.

Once you clean up your body, you may be able to tell an acute reaction to an allergen, by gauging how you feel about thirty minutes after ingesting. If you do not feel good in any way or feeling sleepy, this may be an allergic reaction. If you are feeling funny, or on a high, it may be something not good for you long term.

By monitoring heart rate, blood pressure and temperature, it is possible to detect an allergic reaction. Measure these first thing in the morning, best to do while lying in bed before you get up, write down heart rate, blood pressure and temperature. If you cannot measure blood pressure, just measure temperature and heart rate.

Then eat something or be around something you suspect to have a reaction to, but cannot tell for sure. I have personally found that my heart rate goes UP, my temperature goes UP (or as likely DOWN) and blood pressure goes UP when having an allergic or adverse reaction. The symptoms of a bad reaction may not be the same for everyone. Usually for colds and flu's you get a fever and feel congestion in the head and sinuses.

Allergic reactions can vary. It can be a rash or some internal reaction. I actually had an exotic berry powder drink attack my knee joints, and it took me a long time to figure out that was the cause. It did damage to my right knee and has taken years for it to heal. For any negative health occurrence, consider an allergic or adverse reaction to something.

A simple way to test for adverse reactions is to remove one possible offending item from diet or your environment and see how you feel, then put it back and gauge reaction. If I do not know what it can be, I remove everything I suspect for few days to a week or two, and I add back the most suspected items one at a time.

Often it takes a week or even longer away from an item to tell an acute effect when you bring it back. For instance, you can remove all dairy items from your diet for a week or two, then ingest dairy at a high-level, to see how you feel. If you try this, be careful of acute toxic shock, use professional care. I have activated charcoal capsules on hand just in case. If feeling ill, I take two to four capsules in most cases. I take more if feeling extremely sick, usually about six. No more than ten unless I feel like I am dying.

If I suspect a certain supplement is giving me an adverse reaction. I may remove all supplements and then bring them back one at a time, the most suspect one first. Alternatively, I may remove the most suspected supplement and see how that feels. Remember, a slight reaction may take a few days to build up enough to feel it. I find that I can take a certain supplement for a few days, then it builds up and my kidneys start to hurt. When I stop taking that supplement, it takes a day or two for the pain to go completely away. One may have bad symptoms other than kidney pain that come on slowly and take time to go away once you are off the adverse supplement.

If you think your gluten intolerant, get away from all gluten for a week or two. Then eat a full meal of high gluten filled foods and see how you feel. If you are like me it will feel like a bowling ball is stuck in your gut. To tell an improvement in joint health it may take a month or longer away from gluten to feel a positive effect.

I heard of a woman who was diagnosed as a schizophrenic. The real cause for her illness was an adverse reaction to beet sugar in processed foods. Once she stopped eating beet sugar, she became well. Many illnesses can be due to an allergen, an adverse reaction, to a deficiency, to parasites, or a combination of these

My wife for many years had allergic reactions to many foods, even beans unless they are cooked correctly. She understood she was

allergic to gluten, but only recently found out that she is also allergic to lectin. If she prepares dried beans by changing the water several times while soaking and cooking she can eat them fine. If not, she has painful stomach bloating. She was in her late forties before she knew she was allergic to lectin, neither of us knew before hand that there was such a thing as a lectin allergy. She only found out because she joined an internet forum board about allergies.

The people on the forum board helped her understand her allergy, and how to deal with it. I suggest using such resources to do your own research. For any kind of illness, you should be able to find web sites and forum boards with people who are knowledgeable by direct experience with a condition similar to yours.

Chapter Thirteen

Activated charcoal capsules

If you take two to four activated charcoal pills, this may reduce an allergen toxin and may indicate that it was an allergen. However, this is not hundred percent sure because activated charcoal will also help with food and chemical poisoning.

An example of using activated charcoal, my wife is allergic to some types of dogs, if she pets the dog and rubs her face she can get a migraine. If she takes over the counter pain medicine, it has little effect. However, if she takes two to four activated charcoal capsules, the pain usually goes away in about thirty minutes.

If you are experiencing mild food poisoning, activated charcoal can help clear this up, normally two to four capsules is enough. Activated charcoal does not work for all chemical poisonings so call the poison control center for chemical poisoning, especially caustic poisons. Activated charcoal removes most types of toxins; you should not use it on a regular basis, as it will remove medications and possibly nutrients out of the body. Activated charcoal pills are cheap and can be found in most health food stores and online. The common accepted usage for them in the USA is for hangovers. They are good for far more than just hangovers and I bring them with me everywhere, including vacation trips and hiking.

They can help or cure most any kind of mild poisoning, from bad food, or toxic fumes, help with diarrhea, and help clear up allergic reactions. Activated charcoal is in use for poisoning and drug overdoses in hospital emergency room departments. I have used activated charcoal for good effect in all kinds of mild poisoning events.

Examples: For breathing in too much diesel exhaust, I can remove a headache in thirty minutes with two to four charcoal capsules. For mild diarrhea caused by drinking unclean snowmelt water on a hiking trip, I ended the problem with four activated charcoal capsules. When overseas, many times I became sick from tainted meat, and activated charcoal literally saved me every time.

Another treatment with activated charcoal is to make a poultice, take about two to four activated charcoal capsules. Remove the black powder from inside of the capsule and make a black paste using a little water, and then put this on a wound. It will draw the poison out of the area. Leave it overnight with a clean moist bandage on top.

If in a very acute state of food poisoning, or going that direction you can take about 5 to 10 or more capsules of activated charcoal. The most powerful method in using activated charcoal is to put the black powder from 5 to 10+ capsules into a cup and then poor in boiling water and stir. Let it sit for about one to three minutes, stir and cool down with water. Then stir again and immediately drink while warm. This will put the charcoal into the system the quickest.

Activated charcoal seems to help with breathed in poisonings as well. For any sick feeling due to toxic fumes, I always have a positive effect after taking some charcoal capsules. For snakebite, I would make a poultice and take many activated charcoal pills, depending on the snake and if unable to get to medical care. Of course, seek out medical attention as the first choice as soon as possible. Caution, activated charcoal may interfere with antivenom medication.

If I was out on a camping trip or otherwise unable to get to a doctor and in an acute poisoning situation where I think I may die, I would take a whole bottle of activated charcoal capsules. This is a personal choice, I personally know of no bad side effects from activated charcoal. When traveling and hiking I always carry either a big bottle or a small container of activated charcoal capsules, because they are hard to find in an emergency. I always have a couple bottles at home as well. I cannot count the number of times its use has greatly relieved or prevented a severe illness for my wife, others and me.

A similar, but less powerful remedy is regular tea, especially green tea made hot and strong, this is good for mild food poisoning. Like activated charcoal, it is a good home remedy and on a trip. The best is loose-leaf tea and it is an effective treatment to use charcoal and tea together, this combination sometimes works better than charcoal alone.

For mild food poisoning, you can drink a very strong loose-leaf green tea (my first choice in medicinal tea) or any regular tea. Take four tea bags or equivalent, and make a very strong hot tea. Drink this and keep on drinking strong tea until you feel better. Overseas in the orient, many people drink tea daily with their food. I suspect they partly do so in order to help digest their tainted foods.

I consider normal caffeinated tea to be medication, not a daily drink as it can cause painful crystals in the kidneys for some people. I think this depends on genetics. It seems people from the orient have no trouble drinking tea all their lives. Nevertheless, I gained kidney problems and painful crystals in my kidneys after drinking a good amount of jasmine green tea for about four years. I drank about a quart a day during this period.

An example of green tea for medicinal use; a close friend was sick in the hospital with pneumonia. Intravenous antibiotics cleared up the lungs, but he had painful diarrhea that would not go away. I made an extremely strong loose leaf green tea in a quart thermos. He sipped this slowly, and in twenty-four hours, his stomach problems and diarrhea were gone. I have given strong green tea to others and myself many times for stomach pains, mostly due to tainted foods with good effect every time.

Charcoal is in use as a fecal deodorant for patients with colostomy bags. In spite of the fact that they may take charcoal orally three times daily for years; it has never been demonstrated to nutritionally affect these individuals, who are already at risk of deficiency.

All the evidence I have found shows that activated charcoal is safe to use occasionally when needed for most kinds of poisoning. In addition, my own years of personal experience indicate activated charcoal is safe to use occasionally when needed for mild poisoning events and for mild adverse reactions.

However, charcoal will absorb medication. It may absorb medication given after the charcoal, because it is in the system for a time. For instance if you take activated charcoal capsules and thirty minutes later take medication, the medication is unlikely to work effectively because the activated charcoal may neutralize part of it.

An interesting case, in one animal study, Dr. V. V. Frolkis, a Russian gerontologist, and his colleagues, showed that the lifespan in older laboratory rats increased up to 34% by feeding them charcoal in their diet! (Experimental Gerontology 1984) Toxins, including free radicals, are believed to play a significant role in aging. These toxins will form a stable matrix with charcoal in the gut, and are eliminated from the body.

The researchers thought that the binding up of these toxins in the intestinal tract so they are not re-absorbed into the system is a mechanism that allowed the rats to live longer and healthier. In my personal experience, it seems that the charcoal somehow removes toxins out of the blood system, (breathed in toxins), which may be factor for increasing lifespan.

Chapter fourteen

Heal thyself, while doing no more harm

Often common medicine uses drugs to cover up symptoms of an un-healthy lifestyle. When I say drugs, this includes herbs and homeopathy. Case in point: if people choose to drink alcohol, smoke, eat poorly, and this leads to illness. Then they go to a physician for drugs and surgery. I ask, was it the lack of drugs and surgery that caused the illness? No of course not, but this is what most people do for a cure.

Most often the cause of illness is poor lifestyle choices, for example smoking and eating artery-clogging foods. If you continue with a bad lifestyle after illness, take all the drugs and surgery you can get because it is your only chance.

A better path is finding a health care provider to guide you toward better health habits. To lead you in proper diet and exercise, along with tests and medications and other treatments as needed in the short term. For long-term health, it is best to have clean food and water, sunshine, exercise, rest and a low stress lifestyle. Sadly, once the body fails, it is often impossible to get health back a hundred percent. It is far better not to get in a bad condition in the first place.

Most health crisises are due to preventable

diseases.   If everyone ate well, exercised, and had a decent lifestyle, the health care industry would have very little work, mostly infectious diseases and traumatic care. Much of what modern medicine deals with today are avoidable diseases due to poor lifestyle.

You are in charge of your life, use Biblical Daniel's example in diet and lifestyle to better yourself. The first medicine is food and positive lifestyle. This is preventive medicine, and it can help cure illness. However, once a person is sick it can take a long time to get well by changes in lifestyle and diet. To get well by better lifestyle and diet takes much more effort than just maintaining health. In other words, if a person waits until they are chronically ill before making positive changes, it takes a much stricter effort to regain health.

Often a person who is into health makes mistakes and does things wrong. This is honest. We all make mistakes in life, but be truthful with yourself. If you eat somewhat healthy, but cheat regularly with tasty treats, the good usually does not outweigh the bad. Only the best effort will have success in terms of having a long healthy lifespan. One bad item ingested regularly, no matter if you know it or not may destroy health, even if everything else is perfect.

An extreme example is a person who does most everything perfectly in diet and exercise, but smokes and then gets lung cancer. A more common example is ingesting a harmful item unaware and it is degrading health, such as pesticide from run off inside drinking water.

Therefore, when one goes to a physician it may not improve health and the downhill spiral may only accelerate. Why is that so? Can a physician force a lung cancer patient to quit smoking? He can give them chemotherapy and radiation treatments, so now the patient has cancer, smokes and is having cancer treatments. How healthy does that sound? Years of toxins in the lungs have aged them and burned up their cell divisions.

Many physicians have knowledge of better diet and may help with this process. They should not only push pills and harsh treatment options. Choose your health care provider carefully, shop around, if they have no knowledge of better diet and lifestyle, consider finding another physician. If you are chronically sick never give up hope, keep on trying and researching. Take charge of your life, research health subjects on the internet, find forum groups, and obtain books on health. Pray to God for guidance and for mental impressions about what to do. An impression may come into your mind or help may come in the form of a book, a regular person or a by health care provider etc.

When taking any kind of drug, herb, homeopathy, supplement or medical procedure, do research about it, if not, you may pay for it. Almost all treatments have side effects. Learn about these or risk pain from an unknown side effect. All treatments have percentages of success and failure. Sometimes a treatment is called a success if a patient is symptom free for a number of years, find out their exact definition of success. All tests have a certain percentage of failure. Sometimes these are significant, including false positives for diseases or false negatives for diseases. For instance, there are tests that may give a false positive for AIDS.

As I am writing this book, it is estimated there are more than a half million deaths a year due to counterfeit medications. There are counterfeit medicine producers in India, China and elsewhere for most any kind of medication and supplement. Most of these are sold in third world counties, but could be anywhere. These counterfeits may have non-effective ingredients or worse yet, toxic ingredients. Given the ineffectiveness of governments to deal with this problem to date, it is reasonable to expect this problem to continue into the future. Consider that you may be taking something toxic due to counterfeiting. From one bottle to the next, it may be a different product. Consider the source of your health products and hope they are not knock offs. Watch how you feel as a guide, I personally had a differing effect from one bottle to the next with a certain supplement and stopped taking it.

I cannot count the number of stories I hear about mistakes that doctors and the health care industry make. This is also true in alternative health care. I myself have made mistakes in the past. I have found neutral to bad products in the alternative health supplement market.

Most mistakes I made are due to lack of information. I personally think all products in health food stores should have in depth usage and warning labels on and inside the products. In the USA, they do not because of the law. I would like to see support for knowledgeable usage of supplements.

To be fair, physicians cannot help that people smoke, drink harmful beverages and eat poorly, then come running to them sick because of poor lifestyle. Many people will not change their diet and lifestyle and want a bottle of magic pills. If you want to find a healthcare provider that will be slow to give prescription drugs and have knowledge of diet, exercise and positive lifestyle changes, you will find him or her. If you want drugs, surgery and harsh treatments, you will more easily find it.

An example, a person I know drank about 8-10 cups of coffee a day, had a cup in hand all day long. Then his back started hurting him. He started to run to the chiropractor for back pain and had many treatments, but the pain did not go away! Finally, he and the chiropractor figured out it was mostly kidney pain. Not all the back manipulation in the world would have stopped his pain; he had to reduce the coffee intake. Often kidney pain blends into existing back pain and the sufferer has no idea that the main problem is the kidneys, not the back. Often kidney pain is due to a harmful beverage, herb or a supplement, or allergen food. Anything ingested can be suspect. Not to say supplements or herbs are bad, but a particular person may not be able to handle it.

I am unable to process most vitamin supplements without some kidney pain, but I can take a whole food vitamin at times. I normally do not have back pain so I can tell quickly if I have kidney pain. If a person has existing back pain, the kidney pain may blend into the back pain. It can be tough to tell what is exactly going on, but if you pay close attention, you should be able to tell the difference.

For best health, you should eat the cleanest diet possible and know your body. By this, I mean know what you are allergic too, and know what makes you feel bad. You need to become your own expert in preventative medicine. After all, it is your body, learn what makes it tick, do not depend on others. Genetic differences between people mean differences in what will work for each person. An expert only has direct experience with their own body so they may not know all the variations between people. This is why no expert will have all the answers. All experts are limited by their own finite set of personal experiences.

Western medicine is the best in the world for traumatic injury care and is fair at diagnosis of disease. However, in my opinion, drugs are used too often; they can be toxic and often not a real cure, just a stopgap measure. Of course, sometimes in the short term, strong medications are the only option, but often the real cure for chronic illness is better lifestyle and diet. An approach may be using commercial health care for diagnoses, and then decide what to do next.

The selling of pharmaceuticals, supplements, herbals and homeopathies is profit driven. Surgery may be profit driven and this may cloud decisions in medical care. We could say the same of the alternative health industry, so do careful research. Study any surgical procedure carefully. For instance, does the medical industry in Europe have the same number of mastectomies as in the USA? If not, find out why or risk suffering in ignorance.

Today, we are getting to a critical tipping point. People are ingesting too many bad foods and beverages, so that the average life span in society may reverse. This trend is harming society; many people are unable to function in daily life. In addition, many common measures for illness are treatments that tend to cover up the problem and cause new problems, a never-ending spiral of illness starts. A person of today may be chronically ill coming out of their teens into their twenties and onward, they are sick all their lives. They are mentally and physically sick due to poor lifestyle and diet, unable to function in society. Such a person is a good customer for more treatments, conventional and alternative, but is on the road of never ending ill health.

I expect in the coming years that an excessive cost of health care will breathe new life in preventive medicine. This will encourage a revolution in thought of western society on what to eat and how to do health care. At least I hope this happens, in any case you can take charge of your lifestyle and health.

I myself have no medical care insurance; I have been this way for most of my life. I concentrate on being healthy and on natural cures. Medical care is getting more and more expensive and people have less and less money. Therefore, there is an increasing demand for preventive action to maintain health rather than trying to regain health after illness. Even if health care is available, it is often a pill-pushing mill and those pills will not cure poor lifestyle, so sickness never ends for most people.

Even if I had medical insurance, I would keep my practice in maintaining health by positive lifestyle. I would not take a pharmaceutical unless I really had to and for the shortest possible time. Of course, each person's situation is different. When sick, you should consult with a licensed medical care provider knowledgeable in all options including treatment by lifestyle and diet.

Question; how do surgeons make their money? Of course, by surgery, I am not implying they intend to do unnecessary surgeries, but it is kind of like a metaphor, "The man with a hammer as his only tool sees everything is a nail"! Do your own research before the knife or risk suffering. The best option may be surgery, but do your own homework.

Alternative health also has its strengths and weaknesses. For instance, there are a bewildering variety of gurus and natural treatments, which have different approaches, and some of these are not healthy. Often information in alternative medicine is incomplete or unclear. It seems every health expert, alternative or not, has a different approach.

You must be careful and study broadly, in taking care of your health. First, think about better diet and lifestyle. Then secondarily think about supplements, herbs and chiropractic care and naturopathy medicine. I try to avoid anything manmade especially if new and chemically made, or anything with very strong effect and exotic to me foods. Herbal medicine can be useful for short-term treatment. However, I favor diet and lifestyle as the first choice in medicine, mostly as preventive medicine. This goes along with Biblical Daniel's story.

A knowledgeable health care provider can be a great benefit. If you are really sickly and overweight, a cleansing diet can stress the body even though it is good. I suggest finding a good physician as you need for monitoring. Furthermore, I have found most people who work in health food stores to be knowledgeable. Ask for their help and follow up with more research.

Different health experts have unique ideas on diet. Possible examples are, "The All Raw Foods Diet", "All Fruit Diet", "High Protein Low Carbohydrate Diet", "The Pulse Foods Diet" and "The Vegan Diet", so on.

Whatever guru you follow, you need healthy fats in balance, balance in protein, and balance in carbohydrates. You should have digestible palatable food, and cooked when needed. In general, you want good nutrition, which means all the vitamins and minerals, fatty acids, amino acids and enzymes that your body needs.

A good diet program would strive to have clean foods. By clean I mean little or no preservatives, antibiotics, harmful genetic engineering, toxins, and full of nutrition. Even with different health experts, reasonable sources agree on the major points. Read all sources of information; there are some differences of opinion and grey areas. We all are learning and should never become stagnant. When trying new things; be attuned to your own body, the positive and negative effects. How I feel is my main judge.

There are dangers in some diet practices, if you are vegan or vegetarian then make sure you are getting complete protein and B vitamins. If eating a typical bad American diet, you need to restrict sugar intake, eat less meat, and eat more fruits, vegetables, and greens. You must be careful about not eating exotic (for you) foods, watching for bad reactions that may happen quickly or build up slowly over time.

As people get older, from 20 to 30 and especially 40, and beyond, health tends to go downward. Metabolism slows down, depending on nutrition, and exercise. People find themselves to be overweight and under nourished. If you are sickly, or have symptoms of cramping of muscles anywhere on the body then you are most likely undernourished. A person with chronic fatigue or any other chronic health problem is likely undernourished.

Most people with normal eyesight have a sudden decrease of close up vision at around age forty to forty-five. Few things about getting older are more irritating than losing close up vision. It seems that everything is in small print. I myself had prescription glasses when I was young, however about age sixteen I discovered that I could read and see fine without them and hadn't use them since. The prescribed magnification used for me was minimal. I also found my eyesight became a little stronger without them. My right eye is dominant over my left eye since my teenage years, nevertheless I can see fine.

However, in my late thirties to forties, I started to work in electronics and had to use magnifying visors. My close up vision started to go downhill, as my eyes were adapting to the use of magnification and I am getting older. I again started to use glasses to read, using the inexpensive kind found in drug stores. I noticed this caused my eyes to adapt downward even further to the magnification. My natural vision was becoming weaker for seeing up close. It was a situation of needing the glasses to read, especially very small print, but they seem to be making my eyes weaker.

My father sent me Pinhole glasses. These enable me to read smaller print and books without making my eyesight weaker. They are of an interesting construction as they have little holes in plastic for lenses. When you look through the holes, it has an apparent effect of magnification so you can see a little better. In my experience, they exercise the eyes. I now use them as my primary reading glasses, and my eyes are stronger for it. I find that pinhole glasses are harder use and take a lot of patience. You must want to have stronger eyes verses the convenience of regular glasses. I personally only use these for reading. Of course, everyone's eyes are different so do your own research and experimentation.

In researching the use of Pinhole glasses, you will find differing information from positive to negative. The differences of opinion on both sides are partly due to financial interests. You may want to seek out personal experiences from people you trust. I plan to keep on experimenting with Pinhole glasses as long as I have positive results.

For super nutrition, consider juicing. Juicing is the single most powerful thing you can do for your dietary health. How to juice; first buy a juicing machine; it separates the pulp from the liquid of fruit and vegetables. If you are on a tight budget, juicers can be found in thrift stores. The liquid is loaded with enzymes, vitamins and minerals. Buy most any type of fruit or vegetable you like then juice it and then drink immediately. It is best to avoid strong vegetables such as beets, collard greens or garlic. I will not juice these because they are hard on the stomach. You can replace one meal or snack a day with this juice or add the juice to the meal. This juice is super concentrated in life giving properties, enzymes and vitamins; you can drink far more vegetable and fruit nutrition than you can eat.

Many health experts choose to juice in the morning, because it is convenient. They finish juicing before the hectic day starts and avoid being too tired to juice in the evening, but any time of day will work. Juicing can super charge your body with energy. It is a good way to improve health.

Another method similar to juicing for health is to make a large pot of soup from vegetables, eat the soup, and drink the broth. This is good nutrition, especially when feeling sick. The leafy vegetables will reduce down in size by boiling, so you can ingest a lot of nutrition in this way. When cooking use a large pot, put in salt and healthy oil, use Bragg's amino and nutritional yeast to taste. You need nothing else. Some options for the health soup are garlic, onions and cayenne, add these in, as you desire. I would not go overboard with spices unless needed, for instance garlic and onion for bacterial illness or cayenne for artery clogging problems.

I avoid having too much harsh strong greens such as mustard greens or collard greens. Kale is a good choice for cooked greens; a huge amount of kale will reduce down in size. I use the least amount of water for cooking greens, about three inches of water in a large pot, and roll over the greens into the water as they cook. Cook for about five minutes; eat the greens and drink the water for best health. I find that my old foot and knee injury are better if I get in plenty of greens every week, especially kale.

Most unhealthy people eat excess calories, but need more nutrition. Juicing will put into your body far more nutrition than one can eat with solid food. Juicing preserves all the enzymes and vitamins especially when you drink it immediately. Juice from pasteurized fruit is not as healthy because high heat destroys enzymes and vitamins.

During normal pasteurization, the high heat of boiling kills harmful bacteria, but also destroys enzymes and vitamins. Flash pasteurization by ultraviolet light is a better choice. The best of all is a fresh product or chilled product shipped non-pasteurized. Of course, it must be clean with no pathogens. Nothing compares to fresh homemade vegetable or fruit juice. The nutrition is superior.

Juicing will have an exponential affect on health. In my personal experience, a good clean diet with juicing will turn your life around. Eat as many organic foods as possible; avoid preservatives in diet. Organic foods have no genetic modifications, have few pesticides and are grown in organic fertilizer such as manure, which improves nutrition.

In my personal experience, the reason I made mistakes in health are due to experimentation with new things with a lack of compete information. The biggest danger is trying new things with incomplete information. My health today is great due to my efforts, but along the way, I tried some things that turned out to be harmful. These days I am more aware of my body and pay even closer attention to what is going on inside of me as I experiment. I am cautious in trying out new supplements or exotic to me foods. I am cautious about any kind of new health habit that goes to an extreme. I am cautious of supplements extracted out of nature and concentrated; of chemical manmade supplements, manmade minerals, or any artificial processes that make something that is said to be for health.

I am more open to gentle foods and beverages for health that are natural and not exotic to me. For instance, I am open to real apple cider, remembering that sometimes a food not being unpasteurized adds some risk, but it is usually more nutritious.

I try to be aware of the unknowable, to prevent the unknown from hurting me. Those things that can harm health while unaware are particularly tough to deal with. For instance, something toxic in the water supply can destroy health long before you understand what is going on. I try to be ahead of such dangers by using preventive measures such as filtering tap water with a charcoal filter.

The power of faith, belief and positive thinking

We all have heard of the placebo effect, it is when people are taking sugar pills when sick. Then they become better as if they take a real medicine.

A similar effect may happen with healings tied into faith and religion. A person's belief and faith tied into the assertions of a "healer" may enable them to become well. Sometimes a religious or medical leader will give a person a special item, such as a necklace or bracelet or even a rock. The item is supposed to have special powers. Over time, let us say in a month it somehow helps the person become well.

A question is how to harness the power of human faith in a rational manner, how to use positive thinking in our daily lives? There is a way to do so and gain the results you want out of life and health. It helps if you have a belief in God or a higher power. Here are the daily exercises to tie into the unseen God to better your life.

Every day give thanks for what you have. This can be in the morning, at meal times and during the day when positive things happen for you.

Every day make an effort to be kind to

people, to be honest, to smile at someone, to say a kind word and reduce negative thoughts and actions. Be the kind of person God can be proud of to bless. Every day, think of what you need or like to have in a positive way and reduce negative thoughts.

For example instead of thinking of how sick and weak you feel in a sorrowful way, visualize yourself being well. Close your eyes and imagine yourself doing wonderful physical activities that you enjoy. The same technique for other needs and desires, if you are in debt, instead of dwelling on the debt, visualize earning money and having success from work and business. If you want a romantic relationship, visualize it happening in your mind in a positive way.

Every day look for positive activities that will help toward your goals. Positive thinking and faith for what you need-tied into action is the best way. Some positive activities are praying to God and studying resources about what you need or want, then going to work when good opportunities come your way.

If during the day, you start to feel negative, stop yourself and in a meditative way do this exercise. Visualize that your business and work life will be successful. Visualize that you are active and happy (do not dwell on health problems). Visualize that you live in a wonderful house, have the car you need and a wonderful romantic partner. Visualize going on wonderful excursions and having enough of what you need. Try to feel a real joy while doing these mental exercises as if you are there. One can visualize most anything positive, but it is probably best to visualize what is achievable.

You can write down a list of needs and wants you desire out of life at this point forward, a kind of bucket list. You can make a poster board of these using photos, or draw, or paint these items out.

A problem in many cultures is to consume at the very limit of ability. This tendency puts many people at the edge of financial ruin. It is better to dream about a wonderful, but simple lifestyle within your practical means. Think about a nice lifestyle rather than having big fancy meaningless things of consumption. In your bucket list put in ideas of positive lifestyle, a good life is about how you would like to live. For instance, visualizing having a modest house and car, then going on some low cost relief trips, to see the world and help people in need. Alternatively, think about helping people in your local community.

Be happy and thankful every day when true needs are met. It is a plus if some superfluous desires happen for you as well.

Chapter Fifteen

Preaching on health

Matthew 7:6

"Do not give dogs what is sacred; do not throw your pearls to swine. If you do, they may trample them under their feet, and then turn and tear you to pieces."

There is an information war going on in the health and diet industry and lots of conflicting information. Most of this is due to money interests. At times, you will meet people very sickly. It is best to be gentle when conveying thoughts about treatment alternatives. Most people are not interested about anyone else's helpful ideas and want to live their own way. They will only be offended if you are aggressive in trying to be helpful. After some light probing on your part and only if they seem interested-then gently talk about ideas in alternative health-as long as their interest lasts. Otherwise, just be a happy healthy person and not push ideas in alternative health. (If you are not happy and healthy, it is best to work on your own life anyway)

I myself knew some very sick people that *may* have become better if they went another direction, but my efforts were futile and not appreciated. It is better to be a positive person in a general way and not push ideas about health-when it is not wanted. Remember, if they do not want to hear about it, they certainly will not change. Many people only want magic pills or other magical treatments. To be similar to Biblical Daniel in lifestyle is difficult for most people to understand the benefit, or even imagine doing it.

As you know more about good health practices and feel better, you may want to preach to everyone about your newfound diet and lifestyle. In my long experience, I have found most people are not interested and only will get upset if you try to push health ideas onto them. I have found the best approach is the gentle one at rare times and simply be a positive person. If you are around a person with bad health habits and they are not interested in good health, it is better to leave them alone.

Sometimes, but seldom, a person you meet will be interested, so talk to them. I have found there are many paths of trying to improve health. Therefore, everyone has different ideas, which may or may not be helpful for you. I personally think anyone who is trying to be healthier is on the right path as long as they are not on a really oddball program.

If another health diet program seems strange, just think about it logically. Will it provide carbohydrates, proteins, and fats in acceptable amounts? Will it provide food in a palatable digestible way, and have enough nutrition and calories? If the answers are yes to these questions, then it is not a bad system, just another way.

An example of stark contrast in diet is the Shaolin monks verses native eating Eskimos.

Their diets are drastically different, both with decent to great health as the result. Native Eskimos living traditionally will eat wild fresh meat and fat few people will obtain. They have a long genetic history with this kind of diet. (These days, few Eskimos eat a pure traditional diet, most eat the processed crap as well). Shaolin monks eat a pulse kind of diet; both sets of people are healthy in their environment, although Shaolin monks on average live longer. There are worse diet practices than eating a lot of fresh clean meat. Remember meat in western society is typically not like traditional wild Eskimo meat and animal fat.

Every person has to take in information at their own pace, from the place where they are at today. This is important to understand, because everyone is at a different level in his or her understanding of spirituality, diet and lifestyle.

You will meet people at different levels in health, diet, and spiritual quest. Sometimes it is hard to communicate across the gap. Interests may converge at points, but are different in other aspects. Try to be open, gentle and positive when interacting.

Chapter Sixteen

More on creating a happy lifestyle

Do you hate your job, or have negative people around you, are you a negative person? What are you like? Are you a can't sit still, type "A" aggressive person? If so, then work to become more relaxed. If you are person who cannot seem to get off the couch, try to be more active. Do you have positive active hobbies that enhance health? Alternatively, are your hobbies sedentary, stressful, and not healthy, like smoking a pipe or cigar? Try to find hobbies that are healthy and try to reduce the unhealthy hobbies, strive for balance in life between work and play, exercise and rest.

The best method to find motivation to be healthier is finding a hobby related to physical health. Stress can stop any healthy activity, for instance stress over a sick loved one, over a bad job and poor finances, over a failed relationship. To find a constant hobby in your life which is under your control is beneficial. This hobby, which is positive, can help you through tough times.

The right kind of hobby is part of a direct effort toward a happier lifestyle. For instance, you can take up a goal-orientated sport, like martial arts. At the same time, you can take up a hands on project like woodworking or maybe go back to school. If one hobby or goal does not work out, it is not a failure, just a learning process. Find another positive goal or hobby.

Warning, a positive goal and hobby could turn negative. An example is to run your first marathon; just to finish would be a great achievement! Nevertheless, it would be an unhealthy obsession if this goal totally consumes you. If so, this could lead to problems, such as over training and ignoring work and family. An example is the runner who compulsively runs ten miles a day every day, for many years-a true story. Over the years, he pounded his body too hard, now he is unable to run.

I think running is great exercise, but if too hard on your joints take up bicycling or hill hiking. Hiking hills with a light backpack of around ten pounds, will give plenty of exercise and it is easier on the joints. If physically challenged, try to find gentler exercises. Most local areas have aerobics and swim classes for older or less able people. No matter your condition, have a physical goal to work toward, develop a plan, and train for it every week. For instance, imagine a wonderful trip that you will be able to do once you are stronger!

Try new hobbies or health changes one-step at a time; work on them with small bites. This week try to find a new hobby, or give up bad snack food, and replace it a good snack food. Next week find one new positive friend or social group and limit contact with one negative person. Do not be negative around friends or your social group, even if it kills you! Smile with someone today. Give up a bad habit and start a new hobby, do each positive change in manageable bites.

In life, we may find it hard to change our social economic status, but we always can change our lifestyle. Far more important for happiness is positive lifestyle than social status or money. What your lifestyle should be depends on personality; there is not any single correct lifestyle for everyone. A hard thing to avoid is the ruts we make for ourselves in life. Let others challenge you in a positive way, and challenge yourself with a positive goal, always do new things when you can.

One person may be happy in a situation that would make another miserable. However most people in a positive lifestyle try to be happy no matter their social economic situation and have fun hobbies and activities. They try to have a social network of friends and family that is positive and try to have low stress meaningful work and hobbies. *Happiness is a day-to-day positive habit.* Practice this habit every day.

If life is dealing you rough blows, control what you can. If you are very unhappy in a long-term way, search out alternative methods to fix your mental outlook. If you are unhappy for years do not forget the mind body connection and explore physical causes from allergies, adverse reactions, deficiencies etc. A medical doctor in ecological medicine or a naturopath may be helpful.

Homework, find at least one book about improving happiness and lifestyle and read it. For a month, avoid as much as possible all non-comedy media, in news, books, movies and TV.

Read the funnies in the newspaper, watch comedies on TV, read humorous books (I really like the "Patrick F McManus" series of humorous books). Gauge how this makes you feel after the month and consider keeping this happiness habit.

Chapter Seventeen
Life span, count those cell divisions

When we are born, most of our cells have a certain number of divisions before they die. This number is around fifty divisions before cellular death (information sources vary on the number of divisions before death). When a cell ages, it has two choices when it is worn out. It can die and disappear or it can divide and make two new cells. To continue life, the cell divides and life goes on, but at the end of each cell's DNA there is something called a telomere. These are there to seal off the ends.

After each division, the length of the telomere shortens. At the end of cellular lifespan, the length of the telomere is too short to allow further cell division and instead of division, the cell dies.

People have two ages, a chronological age and a biological age. These are in relation, but not in lockstep with each other. For example, one person at age 60 may have their body broken down; another person at age 75 may be in better condition in terms of overall health and cellular age. If so the 60 year old is biologically older than the 75 year old, how is this so?

Everything in our environment and genetics can effect cellular age and the number of divisions left in cells. Some people have more stress, some people take in more toxins, some people's bodies can handle certain toxins or stressors better and so on. However, no matter your individual genetics you can extend your own healthy life span-if you work on it.

For example, one-person smokes, another does not. Smoking dehydrates the body and the effort to remove the toxin is a strain. The smoker will have less lung capacity to obtain oxygen. The toxins in the cells of the smoker are in a greater strain, as compared to the non-smoker. As you can imagine, the stress on the cells in the smoker's body will age them faster especially in the lungs. At the point of death, each cell has a choice, to die or to divide. It will choose to divide if it can; at that point, there is one less cell division in the cellular lifespan of the lungs.

An imaginary example; a smoker's body cell may divide on average every 1.2 years; the non-smoker may have a cell division every 1.5 years. Therefore, the smoker is biologically older, especially in the lungs, the main area of cellular stress. A person can only live as long as the weakest link in organ health.

Another imaginary example, a woman exercises, and is in good physical shape. Great, exercise is one of the three pillars of health. However, let us say she neglects other areas of her health, will not eat enough nutrition and listen to her body, to let it rest enough. She has a stressful lifestyle. Let us say, she runs a 10K race, and afterward is exhausted and then eats a fast food meal while doing stressful business on a cell phone. After the race, her body's cells are desperate for good nutrition and rest. They are at the edge of living on or dividing to avoid cellular death. Inadequate rest and nutrition puts her body's cells over the edge. Instead of repairing themselves and living on, her cells divide, so there goes another cell division! Stress, excessive exercise, environmental toxins, lack of rest and poor diet all can accelerate cellular aging.

I notice some people, who seem physically gifted, athletic, thin and very active, but still, at some point their body seems to fall apart sooner than it should due to poor lifestyle. This can happen in the thirties on up to the fifties in age. Other people, who from a young age have poor nutrition and lifestyle, are physically falling apart from the beginning. If you are in such a situation, super nutrition, juicing, rest, cleansing and detoxification can help. You need to adopt the best lifestyle possible.

A person needs to have mental awareness of their body, to feel themselves, to know when they need rest and nutrition, when not to push too hard. I personally would not work very long in a toxic work environment without protection. I would walk away. Macho people do not care about their health and do not care about your health. If a company does not care about their workers ingesting toxins, then it will not care when their employees are sick. You should avoid such work situations.

It is common enough for a person to be strong in a toxic environment and ignore bad effects for a while, then pay for it afterward, maybe to the end of life. Examples are numerous, black lung from coal mining, asbestos in lungs, any kind of toxin from chemical fumes and so on. If you are getting sick and cannot obtain adequate protection consider quitting, it is not worth it. A common enough occurrence is painting with toxic paints, such as epoxy paints made for industrial usage. One day of painting without protection will make you sick. Depending on the toxin, permanent damage may take only a few minutes, hours, days or years. It is hard to tell which it will be by feeling the body when it is happening.

During 9/11/2001 terrorist attack in New York City, firefighters went in to help at the trade towers without using enough protection and afterward many became chronically ill. Instead, they needed to follow a plan of using breathing protection and cycling in and out of the area in shifts. This could have saved their health. A person can be strong for a time in a toxic situation and destroy health for a lifetime. It is not worth it. Obtain breathing protection when the lungs start to choke up, demand it. I always use eye protection when I think there is danger of caustic chemicals or an object hitting my face.

Set your mind so if a chemical solution ever did hit your bare face to keep your eyes closed and get to water to flush it out before opening your eyes. Call out to a co-worker and get them to guide you to a water source. Once I had gasoline splash into my face, and I did this technique with good results.

How to protect the cell divisions you have left? Juicing is great. Super nutrition improves health and extends the life span between cell divisions. You cannot gain new cell divisions, but you can extend the life span of the ones you do have. Ingest organic non-processed foods and take food-based vitamins. Do a fasting cleansing program. Get plenty of rest when needed. Arrange a low stress lifestyle. Choose your supplements carefully; avoid harsh chemical effects on organs from bad pills or supplements.

Often parts of the body age at a different rate. An overworked organ may be older than the rest of the body. If you are already in this situation, be extra gentle with your aged organs. Everyone's situation is different about which body parts are more worn out than the rest. Examples are a person with harmed lungs due to industrial toxins and smoking; another with a damaged liver due to drinking alcohol with pills; a third with harmed kidneys due to drinking toxic beverages in excess.

All toxins will age the whole body, but they will age the directly impacted organs the most. In addition, cancer, parasites, and diseases can settle into organ systems that are full of toxins. The human body tries to remove all toxins, but if it cannot it will store them somewhere, often in the body fat in and around organs. This is a place of toxic stress. In this area of the body, there is a lower ability to fight off disease and pathogens. Cancer is more likely to form in a toxin-laden location.

Stress can age you, all three pillars of health, diet, exercise and a happy low stress lifestyle is equally important. Avoid toxins from the environment, not to be paranoid, but be careful and aware. As we get older we want to exercise, but while avoiding injury, sometimes-physical injuries are unrecoverable. Young people do not understand this until it is too late.

If you take up rough sports, do not pound through painful workouts, completely heal up injuries and modify routines as needed. If you choose to be macho now you may pay for it the rest of life. For example, I have a permanent weaker left shoulder due to high school football, a foot in chronic pain that I broke years ago and a weak knee. (All are doing better since I gave up almost all wheat and bread.) I live with these aches while staying active. I recently bought a new book on how to run a marathon. A great achievement that I want to do, but I think it may be too hard for my old knee and foot injuries.

Do not purposely pound your body, you must live in it for a long time, so do not foolishly break it up. Rest when needed, some injuries take many months to heal, maybe years, accept it and do not fight it. You can force yourself to use an injured body too soon. Maybe take a broken bone out of the cast early or start training again too quick. Instead of this, set your mind to extend the recommended rest time by 25%, *trust me.*

Chapter Eighteen

Clean up your environment!

During sleep you want clean air to breathe, I use anti dust mite sheets and pillowcases on my bed. Dust mites bugs live on your skin and eat the dead skin, and get into your bedding; their feces and dead bodies are allergenic. Normal washing does not effectively kill them. They can fill up your mattress and pillows over time. The dust mite sheets block them from getting into your bedding.

When you wash your bedding use borax, this helps to kill dust mites. If you wake up in the morning and feel congested in your nose and sinuses, this may mean you are breathing in something toxic overnight. Things to check for are pets sleeping with you, mold, dust mites and fumes off bedding. I always have an air filter system in my bedroom. The most convenient kind is those that you can clean out the filter yourself. If too noisy at night just run it during the day to clean the bedroom air, in addition you can open a window during the day for cleaner air.

I once got new 2.5-inch memory foam top for the bed; I was sick every morning from breathing the fumes off it. I had to get rid of it, to the dismay of my wife. Later on, we obtained a ten-year-old memory foam top for the bed that I can use. The fumes off old glue and plastic products are much less.

Breathing in fumes and dust from anything can erode health; watch out for chemical fumes and any sort of dust while working. I do carpenter work at times and I try to be careful and not breathe in wood dust while sawing and working. The worst seems to be manmade wood products with glue in them. Have you ever noticed a strong chemical smell from new construction? It is chemical fumes off the building products. If you are sensitive, it may be better to live in an older home and use older building products or choose natural building products. Use natural wood and masonry over plastics and glue filled wood products. I try to be careful with paint fumes and use a respirator. I recently used a spray product to waterproof some of my hiking clothing and it was harsh on my lungs, next time I will use a respirator.

To avoid chlorine inside treated water use a shower filter and a water filter, these are inexpensively found in local hardware stores. My wife found that her hair seems better when using a filter on the shower.

I use eye protection; we only have two eyes and cannot replace them. It only takes a second of good sense and not suffer for the rest of life. If you look at most accidents, in most instances a brief mental mistake happened, a bad choice made in a few seconds. Do not be flippant with your choices in life and work. Metal structures often fail quickly without warning-metal collapse can happen in an instant. Wood structures usually give a warning with buckling and crackling sounds.

I am not worried about low levels of

electromagnetic radiation, but I am cautious about living near a large transformer. The strength of electrometric energy falls off by the inverse radius squared equation ($1/r^2$). So if you move twice as far away, the radiation is four times weaker; if three times the distance, it is nine times weaker; if four times the distance, then sixteen times weaker. Therefore, a farther distance away usually means a great reduction of radiated energy. Still, one has to be careful of focused beams of energy such as from microwave antennas. If you are worried about cell phones or other small electronic devices, carry them in a backpack or purse or lay them a short distance away from you. Use them a little distance away from the face. The little bit of added distance will greatly reduce any possible harm. For an electric blanket, use it to warm up the bed and turn it off.

When working, a few protection items are important. Always bring work gloves, rags, dust masks, eye protection, and a quality respirator. Use heavy rubber gloves for chemicals. You will have personal protection if you bring these items to any job site,

Chapter Nineteen

Competitive mentality verses adaptive mentality

The western culture puts emphasis on being strong, tough, to exercise hard to gain strength. However, there is a gaping hole in western culture in terms of how to go about being healthy, about how to read the body in its current condition, and then decide what to do next.

Even sports performance can suffer from lack of balance in popular culture. To be stronger means to work out hard, but there is little about how to adapt and blend into environment. People often do not know how to exercise gentler when needed, to rest and recover. To seek out the best diet and avoid adverse reactions to foods, supplements and environmental items.

Western people have a desire to play football in the evening, and then go out at night drinking beer and eating hot wings. In youth, this may work for a few years, but it is a drain. This kind of activity will use up cell divisions at a faster rate.

People should know that to eat well and rest is to be healthy, and this will translate to strength and endurance-especially in older years. Meat and potatoes are a common meal, with a dash of greens for good measure. What if this meal with a bit of greens is not nutritious enough? Chronic weakness and illness will set in when you exercise heavily and the body cannot support the effort anymore. A person can mentally force their body onward too long until physical breakdown sets in.

For instance, in the common bad USA diet there is a high volume of fats and carbohydrates and proteins, but not enough nutrition to provide all needed vitamins and minerals. The food calories are from processed foods and are often toxic. To eat enough nutrition takes a conscious effort in western culture. To eat enough fruits, vegetables and greens every day takes extra effort in modern society. Make it a habit to eat raw fruits, raw nuts, raw seeds, raw or lightly cooked vegetables for snacks and even for meals. It is best to drink clean water as the primary beverage.

Learn how to feel your muscles, know when you are ready for more exercise or needing rest. If you are on an exercise schedule, let us say three workouts a week, before the next workout squeeze and contract the muscles, use full range of motion. If you are more than a little sore, then you may need more time to recover and more protein and nutrition. You may decide to do a light workout, only to get the blood and lymph fluid moving,

Exercise only makes you more fit in the recovery phase. Exercise tears the body down; afterward only good nutrition and rest allow recovery to a stronger condition. If rest and nutrition are inadequate, then the muscles are torn down again before they are repaired. Growth can be less than it could be, or strength goes backward.

Having a mind-body connection is important. Do not blindly follow a workout program, feel the body. Most exercise programs have a set number of workouts per week and a certain amount of time per workout and so on. Follow any suggested program by how you feel. I can lift weights in my forties. Currently I have been doing so only once a week, and in addition, I am rock climbing once a week and this is enough. I am always varying my workouts and hobbies to keep up interest. I may be doing something different next year.

As exercise increases, your nutrition and calorie needs increase. Let your mind-body connection be the guide. If you want to lose weight, you need to feel a little hungry, but if you are starting to feel lethargic and weak then you need more rest, calories and nutrition. If you go into a new workout session with sore muscles, how sore are they? Did you have enough rest, nutrition and protein, should you rest another day or not? If you are very sore, this means you do not have full recovery. When people exercise and diet at the same time with enough nutrition, they convert fat into muscle. Most people are deficient in nutrition to varying degrees. Very common deficiencies are lack of potassium, magnesium and calcium.

Dieting without exercise leads to failure in terms of good health. In such a program, you may be turning into a thinner person, while losing muscle. Often people stop dieting and then regain the fat and more, but not the muscle. A few cycles of failure like this and you are a sick fat blob with less muscle than when starting out!

In addition, metabolism becomes slower than when starting out.

A better approach is to have some kind of weight bearing strengthening exercises and aerobic exercises on a regular basis along with good nutrition and diet. Have your diet program tied into a physical hobby with goals and positive lifestyle. Dieting while keeping a poor lifestyle will not work very well. Vary your program over time as needed to keep it interesting, this is an approach to have a lifelong positive lifestyle.

What is a negative verses positive lifestyle you may wonder? A negative lifestyle is living a sedentary life, with unhealthy hobbies such as smoking, drinking, gambling and running around aimlessly. Another example of a bad lifestyle is poor diet, smoking and drinking while excessively working. Alternatively, a positive lifestyle is balancing work with play. To have a variety of hobbies and activities that is both physically and mentally challenging, and fun. Each person has a different personality so a positive lifestyle for one person may not work for another. In general, positive lifestyle is a clean healthy way of living with good diet and exercise. To have positive social interactions with other people and balancing work with play, most of us can always better our lifestyle. Always try new activities that make life interesting, this does not have to take a lot of money, for instance you can learn to play the guitar.

A positive way to approach exercise and sports is to be less competitive with others and less willing to push yourself when feeling bad. Be more adaptive, flowing with your day-to-day physical rhythms. If you feel strong, go for a hard workout. If you feel weak, do less, rest and eat good nutrition.

If you are physically pounded by a hard workweek, maybe it is time to rest up and lie in the sun, rather than be a weekend warrior. Try some juicing, eat a big pot of cooked greens, and have some raw fruit. If emotionally stressed out, this can cause you to feel tired. If so, it is often best to do a physical workout to feel better.

Develop a mind-body connection; think about how to heal thyself. (If your subconscious thinks something will hurt you, it most likely will).

Do not ignore what your body is telling you, I have had cramping legs and feet in the past. I suspected this to be a lack of something, and eventually found out it is a lack of electrolytes, which I can treat short term by salt, sport powders and sports drinks. However, these are the not the best long term remedies as they hurt my kidneys. I then found a food-based supplement that had magnesium, potassium and calcium in it that I took along with extra salt. This helped some. Finally, I started to eat more greens and raw nuts and seeds, which is the natural solution. This was the best and final solution, because I was able to cut down on salt to a minimum amount, which is better for my kidneys and blood pressure.

What I did was search on the internet. I looked for the likely causes for cramping, and then I took action while feeling my body to see what worked best. Of course, to see the right kind of doctor for tests is a good approach, if you have insurance or can afford it out of pocket.

The best source for nutrition and minerals is from food, organic greens, fruits, and vegetables, but it may be hard to buy enough if on a budget. I started my own greens garden and I am thinking of a small green house in the future. I personally prefer getting all nutrition from foods for the least possible damage to organs. This is best for long-term health.

What physical or even mental problems do you have? They are symptoms; usually there is a cure if you seek it out. Muscle cramping was a mineral electrolyte problem for me, which I solved. I cannot say every health problem is curable by diet and nutrition, but I believe most chronic health problems have a natural cure.

The puzzle is figuring out the cause of the illness and finding a natural way to treat it gently and effectively. In my experience, you must be relentless in your search and not give up. It can take days, months, even longer to figure out what is going on and know what to do. Often the cure is taking out something harmful out of the diet or environment or adding something in and having better lifestyle.

Chapter Twenty
Solving your illness problem

First is a list of causes for illnesses, and possible treatments.

1) Viruses: Avoid sick people and risky practices such as unprotected sex and needle sharing. Proper diet and lifestyle will boost the immune system, which is your best first defense. Some at home, treatments are high dosages of vitamin C, herbs, sunlight, fresh air, ionic and colloidal silver, wheat grass, and homeopathies.

2) Bacteria: Try to avoid sick people because some communicable diseases are deadly. Many people in a weak condition go to the hospital, catch something like pneumonia, and die. The best defense is positive lifestyle and good diet for a strong immune system. Some at home, treatments are high dosages of vitamin C, herbs, sunlight, and fresh air, ionic and colloidal silver, wheat grass, and homeopathies.

3) Parasites: These can enter your system from food (undercooked meat), feces, from dirt when crawling around as a child, from pets, and from untreated or unfiltered water. They may be in the body for years and when the immune system becomes weak from toxins or age, they can rise up to cause acute illness. As prevention, cook meat thoroughly, treat and filter water, wash hands after petting animals and worm pets regularly. A simple preventive action is to do a parasite cleanse every year or so by using certain herbs. Taking a combination of wormwood, cloves and black walnut hulls can work. In addition, other herbs and spices are antiparasitic.

4) Toxins: In daily life, we ingest toxins all the time and the body tries to remove them. If it cannot, the body will store these toxins somewhere, possibly in the fat around organs. In the modern world, the amount of ingested toxins can be very high, from food additives, toxic fumes in industry, home products and the environment. One can take activated charcoal for an acute ingestion of a toxin. Another method is fasting to clean toxins out of the body. There are chelating treatments that will remove toxins out of the body and organ systems. The chelating chemical will attach itself to the toxin so it can be removed. A common chelating intravenous treatment is in use to remove toxins out of clogged arteries for heart patients. Natural chelating agents are fresh greens and green powders such as wheat grass, oat grass and spirulina, all of these are good supplements. (Remember, a needed mineral or vitamin can be ingested at a too great amount and then become toxic in time.)

5) Deficiencies: It is best to eat a balanced diet, full of raw or lightly cooked organic vegetables and fruits. Most people become deficient due to eating too much processed foods full of sugars and grains. The heat of pasteurization destroys vitamins and enzymes in common foods. In modern life, we have gone too far away from the intended natural diet, which gave nutrients from simple foods. It is difficult for people to obtain all needed nutrients because of eating processed foods. Even people into being healthy are often not getting enough nutrition. Supplementation is an option, but harsh supplements may damage organs over a long time. I suggest eating raw or lightly cooked foods every day; such as vegetables, fruits, nuts, seeds, and plenty of organic greens. Fermented and sprouted foods are very nutritious as well. It takes an extra-unaccustomed effort for most people to obtain all needed nutrition from food.

6) Stress: Even if everything else is perfect in life, stress can hurt health and lifespan. Stress releases hormones, which puts people into a never-ending flight or fight state of emotion. Food does not digest when in this condition and then becomes toxic in the stomach and intestines. Often extreme stress is because of abusive family members and the inability of a person to control their life. The first step is usually getting away from stressful situations and people, and working toward emotional and financial independence. If stress at work is too much, develop a plan to move toward better employment. Find books and other resources to study about improving your particular situation.

7) **Poor lifestyle**: What is poor lifestyle? There can be varying opinions, but I would consider it to be eating unhealthy, lack of exercise, lack of positive hobbies and a lack of balance in life. Not mixing work and play in a positive way, not having time to rest and enjoy life. Being negative rather than positive, having bad habits, dreaming of wealth and owning things rather than having a balance in spiritual life. Most people learn their lifestyle from their parents and peers from an early age and never grow up as a person. To change, take stock of your lifestyle today and start to study everything you can about the subject of better lifestyle, philosophy, and better health. Often a person needs a hobby to help improve other parts of life, like a sports hobby, or the right kind of social group. Do not let the new hobby be negative or stressful, if it becomes stressful then make another change.

8) **Poor diet**: Most people learn how to eat from an early age with very little consideration about how to be healthy. It is hard to change poor diet habits to better ones. To eat healthy may be a strange concept for some people. They may be adapted to a bad diet due to family habits and popular culture, but it seems normal to them so they think it healthy enough. It is best to study the subject of eating better as widely as possible and to make changes slowly, and experiment on new ways of diet and food. If one makes an honest effort and keeps on growing, they are on the right path.

9) Adverse reactions or allergies: It is possible to eat something that makes you very sick that others can eat safely. Everyone is different, but family traits are passed down every generation or every other generation. If grandma had migraines all her life, you may have them too, if you do not understand why and work to prevent them. In today's world, there are countless additives and exotic out of area foods to consume and these are changing all the time. You must identify and eliminate harmful items to maintain health. For instance, GMO and additives can change foods from one year to the next. Understand food addiction, often a person is addicted to a food that causes adverse reactions.

The first step for better health is a parasite cleanse. Go to a health food store and they will help you find an anti parasite formula. I personally like a product with these herbs, cloves, black walnut, and wormwood. In capsule or tincture form, I take the prescribed dosage on the bottle or what is recommended by separate literature until the bottle is empty. I normally do a parasite removal program every year to two.

Most people think de-worming humans is a strange idea, but we all do so for our animals. Should not parents de-worm their children who craw around on the ground since babies? I ask the reader, have you ever done a parasite cleanse in your whole life? What are the odds of getting parasites over the years from the ground, pets and under cooked meat? A parasite infection will erode health and the effect increases with age because toxins have built up in the body and the immune system is weaker. A weak immune system is less able to fight off parasites. It is possible to have parasites and not know it. You may not have strong enough symptoms to know that ill health is because of parasites.

For myself, I consider a parasite cleanse a basic first step in working toward better health. If during a treatment no parasites are removed, then no matter, because no harm is done. Watch out for an adverse reaction to the parasite treatment herbs being used. If you are full of parasites, you may feel slightly sick during treatment, this is normal.

Another parasite treatment is using a "Bug zapper". It is an odd concept that most will not accept, but I will include it in this book for completeness. If one is chronically ill, then using a "Bug zapper" is an option. It is an electronic device that produces a DC pulse at 50 to 500,000 hertz at 5 to 10 volts. You take the two handles of the zapper in your hands and do three treatments for about 7 minutes each at around 5 to 10 minute intervals. The shocks are said to kill harmful bacteria, viruses and parasites. It is said that it will kill these in the body, but not in the stomach and intestines. I have done this treatment, and frankly, I could not tell if it actually worked or not. However, I feel it is harmless to try, as the shocks are very slight. It may be worth a try if you are chronically sick, do your own research. My resource is the book: "The Cure for All Diseases". by Hulda Clark. You can find more information on the internet.

A common deadly affliction is pneumonia. Anyone with a weak immune system is likely to die from it, especially older people. Anyone with pneumonia symptoms must be taken to a doctor right away. These are shaking, chills, fever, chest pain, abdominal pain, cough and general feeling of extreme sickness. Sadly, in recent years we have the rise of pneumonia super bugs that are antibiotic resistant. In the future, the most likely deadly epidemics are those from air born diseases, possibly something similar to pneumonia. The best at home treatment that I know of is using a nebulizer with a powerful medication. A nebulizer puts water into a mist, into which you can add medicine to breathe into the lungs. Possibilities are ionic or colloidal silvers or iodine made for this use. If one wants to prepare for a possible pandemic or pneumonia, a nebulizer with medications is an option, maybe the best one.

In addition, my wife treated her father when sick with pneumonia by using water treatments, called fomentations. About four times a day she would place hot wet towels on the chest, then remove, and wipe down the chest with cold wet cloths. This is a method to force the water out of the lungs and to boost white blood cells. There are many effective water treatments and they are remarkable for their effectiveness, simplicity and low cost. In today's modern world of super bugs, which are resistant to antibiotics, one may want to become familiar with such techniques. In addition, modern medicine has become unaffordable for many people. A good resource for water treatments is "The Natural Remedies Encyclopedia" by Vance H. Ferrell and Harold M.

Cherne, MD.

Further steps for health: I may take a good food based vitamin complex when I think I need it. Depending on symptoms, I may get some other supplements. I suggest when starting out to consider taking a high dosage of a balanced vitamin complex for a short time, especially if you have chronic health problems. Long-term, I think it is best to transition toward getting all needed nutrition from foods while using little supplementation.

Why strive for the least amount of supplementation-for the healthiest program? Let us look at three sets of people who live in a natural way in the mountains. Vilcabamba, who live in Ecuador's Andes mountains; Hunza, who live in the high mountain regions of Pakistan; Abkhasia, the ancient peoples in the Caucasus in southern Russia. All these people have a long healthy lifespan, where diseases and debilitation are rare. Many live past a hundred years in good health, some live even longer, up to 130 years. They do so in a low stress, happy lifestyle, with no supplements. They eat natural whole foods, and drink clean mountain water. They are a rich people in life, but poor in material wealth. I think they have a stronger connection to God than most western peoples.

Vaccines: There is a lot of controversy about vaccines. I lean toward avoiding them. If you get a vaccine, ask for the non-mercury kind. In addition, you can take a dosage of activated charcoal before and after the vaccine to help remove any possible toxins. You can make a homemade activated charcoal poultice and put it on the place of the vaccine shot and it will draw out any possible toxins. In addition, charcoal poultice patches are available in some health stores and on the internet.

One does not have to live in an isolated mountain village for long life and health. However, it takes more discipline in the modern world. Some people in the west have a long healthy lifespan, but it is the exception. It is important for parents to start children off right and teach them the healthiest ways. Children should know the reasons why they need a health diet program. Nevertheless, I think parents should allow children processed treats at rare times, selecting the healthiest forms because for no other reason children may rebel later on in life. A child should not suffer at a birthday party in a friend's house-unable to eat any of the cake and ice cream, or is unable to go because something there may be harmful. Such social eating events at great intervals will not harm health.

All these suggestions are the first steps toward fixing health. Start to think about juicing vegetables, obtain any bright colored organic vegetables and juice them, like kale, spinach, and swiss chard. Healthy green powders are barley grass, wheat grass, oat grass, spirulina, kelp and others, all are good choices for better health. We once had an old crippled dog that came back to life for a while when we fed her green powders.

You need to consider foods that may cause an allergic reaction or are unclean. For health, the best foods are those you prepare yourself from an organic, non-GMO source. Bad health may be due to foods, beverages, or environmental toxins. A method is to study recommended diets for health and then clean up your diet as much as possible. Then experiment by taking items away from your diet and add them back in, while judging how you feel when making changes. In experimentation, you should be adding and removing healthy food items, but possibly not for you due to individual genetics. For example, most people can eat the vegetables in the nightshade family, but for some people it may trigger an arthritis attack.

Poor health for many people is a chronic condition due to failure of diet, exercise and lifestyle. Baring physical injury or genetics, most illnesses are because of poor lifestyle choices. Ordinary medical care is great for diagnosis some of the time and may come up with treatments for acute illness caused by parasites, viruses, bacteria, and physical injury. Sometimes surgery is necessary, but always gets a second and third opinion. For chronic illnesses due to bad lifestyle, the real cure better lifestyle.

There is no pill to cure the bad effect of an allergen food, or unhealthy eating, or a pill to make you exercise. Therefore, many chronic illnesses are only in your own power to cure or at least make better. Common medicine can be a good choice to diagnose health problems. However, I would be cautious about a diagnosis that seems to need a pill forever and never has a real cure. For this diagnosis, I would consider restarting my search for the cause of the illness, studying my diet and environment first.

If you have a chronic illness, it can be

caused by one or many identifiable causes. If so, you can cure yourself or greatly improve your situation, and not mask the problem with a treatment (pill) that may cause other illness because of side effects.   If a doctor is not knowledgeable about diet, parasites, and adverse reactions to foods, allergens and heavy metal toxicity, and about causes of illness that have real final cures, then find another one.

Often a person is pushed through a pill-pushing dispensary, called modern medical care. This book is written for people all across the world, of which many are poor. If this is your situation, try to find a lower costing medical care practitioner. The money spent is well worth it, but if unable, then you are left to your own devices. Read resources on health and find health food stores. Remember, there are bad products out there even in the alternative health arena. Sadly, written testimonials are not a certain guide, as they can be made up. It is better to find a personal testimonial directly from someone you trust.

Of course, if the only solution for chronic health problems is pharmaceuticals then of course take them long as needed. Nevertheless, I suggest never stop looking for a method that leads to a final cure.

If you are sickly and traveling, do not go from a first world country to a third world country! Find out the common diseases and afflictions in a area before you go. Now is the time to pack your travel medicine chest. You should have what is needed for the most likely diseases, in herbs, supplements, and homeopathies, etc. You may or may not want to be vaccinated, a personal choice. I would carry a lot of activated charcoal, a parasite cleanse formula, iodine to treat water and intestines, and a water filtration system. One can drink water with a little iodine in it to treat infected intestines and it may help. Buy tea when in country. I think the best tea for medicine is loose-leaf green tea.

In my experience while being overseas in Central Asia, tainted meat is the biggest danger. I got sick many times from slightly rotten meat and in every instance-activated charcoal saved me. I never had problems with water or fruit, but I have not traveled that broadly in the third world. In third world countries, meat is often sold in open air with no refrigeration. The cheapest meat is likely to be slightly rotten. A common situation is that you are with poor people who feed you meat that is tainted, and since it is a social situation, it is next to impossible to refuse. Drink all the tea they offer and be ready with activated charcoal, take a lot if getting sick, at least 5 capsules, to 10 and more. Good luck, diarrhea kills more people than anything else in the world. When traveling to a foreign country, especially into third world tropical areas you are risking catching something that will harm health the rest of life.

The biggest danger for someone traveling from the third world to first world is due to eating rich processed foods. They should resist junk foods and stick to their accustomed diet-if it is healthy.

Supplements, even the best ones are processed. The worst can be harsh on your body. When seeking out alternative medicine, I am careful about exotically caused illnesses, which of course need exotic treatments. I believe most of the time illnesses are due to poor diet and adverse reactions and all you need is a simple method of action.

The trick is figuring out what is wrong and acting correctly. If you are unwilling to quit smoking or eating fatty pork products or give up an addictive allergen food, then it will be impossible to cure chronic illness. I have found many people think they are eating healthy, but they are making serious mistakes.

Another personal example: In my late twenties to early thirties, I had chest pains from my heart. I ignored it, but I was concerned. My Dad who is a wide reader told me to stop eating anything with hydrogenated oil in it. I then noticed that if I ate foods with a lot of this oil, I would have chest pains.

I stopped eating anything with hydrogenated oil, which is inside many packaged foods, and my chest pains mostly went away. This is good, as my family on my Dad's side has a long history of early heart attacks and my Dad had a heart attack in his fifties. Luckily, I escaped this fate thus far, by being careful about bad fats and oils, and limiting sugar intake. I plan to avoid a heart attack, as I get older. A heart attack may destroy the capacity to pump blood-carrying oxygen and may cripple a person aerobically for the rest of life.

Hydrogenated oil is oil that has hydrogen put into it under pressure and heat. This makes it into a hard to digest oil. Depending on genetics, it may destroy health. I know of some people who eat quite a bit of this oil and it seems not to affect them. For me, I am sure I would have had a heart attack if I had not stopped eating it

Biblical Daniel and his companions were young Jews taken from their homeland. They were forced by the king to be in the city-state Babylon (located in present day Iraq), and made to study the king's language and other lessons for the service of the King. As part of this, they were required to eat from the King's Table, which had excess meat and wine, to sustain them in their living and studying.

To Daniel, the King's meat and wine were part of the king's worship of idols, of which he could not take part. In addition, the food was from unclean origins, possibly pork or other unclean scavenger meats. His faith would not allow him to eat the King's meat. The boss over the eunuchs allowed their simple diet only after Daniel showed he was better without it.   Therefore, Daniel and his companions studied hard for three years and kept their clean diet. They received a blessing from God.

What does this lesson mean for you? What it means to me is that controlling diet in the right way is part of a positive lifestyle.

It is not a punishment from God if you cannot control your appetite. In fact, you are punishing yourself. It is so easy to eat in excess the fatty, sweet, and processed foods. Especially in the modern world of easy access to unhealthy food, it takes knowledge and discipline to be healthy.

Daniel and his companions ate better, lived cleaner, and thereby kept their minds and bodies clear even with a danger from the King. They also studied diligently and used their time in a productive way. They did the best they could with their situation.

Most people fail to control their appetite, lust and other carnal feelings in life. This can lead to personal ruin. If you choose to work toward personal discipline and have a positive core belief system that you adhere to, life will have more meaning and purpose. We all have a purpose in life, no matter how small or large. Daniel and his companions paid special attention to the small details in their work life.

Some people wait for a big special event in their lives to show how important they are. It is a different approach in trying to do a good job with all the small details. Even the menial tasks are important and the sum of these actions builds together to a whole, showing good character. Daniel and his companions focused on being excellent even in the daily mundane tasks.

After three years of study and healthy lifestyle, Daniel and his companions were ten times above all the rest in the King's realm. This means that you can be healthier, happy and stronger following Biblical Daniel's example. Even more intelligent if you improve your diet, lifestyle, and have a solid moral grounding to live by. Over time because of their positive clean lifestyle and moral faith, Daniel and his companions became leaders in the King's realm.

If you ask God, your higher power to help

you to be on the correct path, I believe that you will be healthier and stronger than most, just like Biblical Daniel and his companions. Material wealth can be fleeting and hollow. Of far much greater value is moral and spiritual wealth. The humble blessed person is rich without material wealth. The richness is in being happy and healthy. What wealthy person would not give it all away for more years of living in perfect health?

Nothing can be as frightening as having a serious illness with an unknown cause. Let us create an example, such as chronic bloating and abdominal pain. Look to find the most knowledgeable doctor you can and be choosy because some health practitioners are not that good. Pray to God and wait for an impression that is reasonable and helpful. However, you must do your part, and read every resource on health that you can find. It is important to have knowledge from many resources. Find further information on the internet and even join discussion forums with people who have similar health problems.

In some instances, illness is due to a mechanical problem, such as bad genetics. Perhaps you are born with a bad heart valve, if so, little can be done on your own without surgery, but one can try anyway with research and God. If it is a virus or bacterial illness, there are conventional and natural treatments to boost the immune system and kill the pathogens. For example, use colloidal silver or short-term high doses of vitamin C. When chronically sick always consider parasites and do an herbal parasite cleanse.

In my own experience, the acute illnesses that can be best tackled by the individual are those that are due to adverse reactions or allergic reactions to something ingested or in the environment. The kinds of chronic health problems, which are easiest self-curable, are those because of bad foods, drinks, and environmental toxins that make people sick due to over ingestion. Illnesses due to lack of complete nutrition are also self curable.

Another personal example: I remember having nosebleeds at times in my twenties to early thirties. Years later, I figured out that these were caused by high blood pressure due to an adverse reaction to certain kinds of red fruits or vegetables, such as beets or boysenberry juice. I now understand what is going on. Today, I know how to better deduce such bad events, by knowing there must be a cause to create the effect of nosebleeds. That it is likely because of something I breathed in, touched, drank or ate, etc.

When sick I know how to think about finding the cause and effect relationship, to pay attention to everything in my daily life. Most people do not notice cause and effect when they feel sick. Therefore, illness will continue and become more acute in time. One should pay attention to what they ate and drank during the day and what chemicals they are around, to remember everything.

Every morning when you get up you should feel good. If not, most likely you did something wrong the day before, if you feel good then you did right. For instance, if I get up feeling rough most likely it is because of something bad I ate the night before. If I feel good then most likely I ate correctly and had no late night snacks. Pay attention to how you feel every morning-while reflecting on the past. If you feel rough first thing, in the morning then likely you have room to be healthier, up to ten times as like Biblical Daniel.

Relief from an illness is often by a very simple action. However, to find a cure may take a relentless search over days, weeks to months. I do not believe people get ill for unknowable reasons. I believe there is a simple cure in most cases. This has been the experience for me in my life.

Example: Clogged arteries are causing chest pains. I know a simple cure is to clean up my diet and or fasting, if I have the willpower.

(We are assuming here that clogged arteries are the only cause of chest pains, which is not true. This is where professional diagnosis may be important).

Example: I have the feeling to go number two in the bathroom, but am unable.

Acute or chronic constipation is no joke. It is probably due to something you ate recently or regularly. Long-term treatment is changing diet, pills, and supplements toward what your body can digest. Obtain more healthy fiber in the diet as well. For acute problems, one can take a laxative or an enema. Stuck feces in intestines can make you sick and cause kidney and or liver pain. If this is the case, an enema can bring relief quickly.

Example: I have a migraine headache. By paying attention, I understand it is an adverse reaction to chemicals in a lotion on my face and or an allergic reaction to a pet.

Treatment is simple, elimination testing.

Example: I have muscle cramps in my toes and legs.

By research and thought, we understand a simple cure may be ingesting essential minerals (electrolytes) such as salt, magnesium, calcium, and potassium. Either by using supplementation or by eating foods that are nutritious in what is needed. The best long-term solution is to eat foods that are more nutritious.

Example: I have chronic clogging in my nose and sinuses, especially in the mornings.

This symptom can have many causes, such as allergens or toxins in the air, or bacterial or viral infections, or may be a combination of all of these. The first step is to check the environment, especially in the bedroom and bed. To clean up the air buy an air filter. Open a window during the day to air out the room. You may use a dehumidifier or humidifier. You can use dust mite covers on the bed and think about how to boost the immune system. You may use a netti pot to wash out sinus congestion. Sometimes, in extreme cases of allergies and breathing problems, you may move to a new house or even to a different part of the country. Think about testing this by going to a new location for a time. Other possible treatments are herbs and ionic silver sprays up in the nose. Bacterial infections of the sinuses are particularly hard to get rid of. Get professional help if needed. Chronic sinus infections may happen due to swimming in water infested with aggressive bacteria (untreated sewage in water).

Example: I am having painful bloating in my intestinal area, an enema gives great relief but I do not know what is wrong.

The first step is thinking back to what you have been eating in the last few days to weeks. Many people find that they cannot digest grains or foods made of grains very well due to gluten, lectin, yeast, proteins, mold, additives or some other reason. Understand if you have adverse reaction to one type of grain, it is very possible you will have problems with others. The gut is made to digest difficult foods so it is not very sensitive to send you pain signals. Thus, it may be difficult to feel when an adverse reaction begins. You must pay close attention to how you feel in the gut area and notice any other signs of adverse reaction. Signs are itchy sensations or a rash anywhere on the body, or a swollen belly and intestine area.

There are countless allergies; the best procedure is to do research on the internet about your particular situation. There are many people on forums that can help and it is likely some will have similar problems as you. Seeing the right kind of medical care professional is a good idea, especially for children. A blanket approach is not to eat anything that is similar to what you are allergic to in any amount. You can also grow sprouts; ferment foods, and soak beans or grains before cooking to make them easier to digest. See: "The Maker's Diet" Jordan S. Rubin.

Modern agriculture grows grains that may be hard for some people to digest because human history with some of these is short. As people age, bad reactions tend to increase and nutritional uptake diminishes because the digestion system is getting weaker.

Example: I notice that after I drink dairy milk I have stomach pain, bloating and phlegm (commonly called flem that causes throat clearing). I also notice that I do not feel well after eating cream or ice cream.

Since most adults cannot digest dairy we know you are having an adverse reaction to dairy. It is common for people to be lactose intolerant and the milk protein casein in dairy is unhealthy in concentration and may cause an allergic reaction. You can experiment with yogurt, cheese, cottage cheese and butter to see how you feel when eating these. Signs of slight adverse reaction to dairy products are chronic sinus clogging and phlegm. In addition, if you eat a lot of cheese at one sitting you may feel clogging in the arteries and veins. It is well known that casein protein is a cancer-causing agent. About 80% of milk protein is made up of casein.

Casein is used as a food additive and is inside many processed food products.

Example: I feel rough in the morning, kind of hung over, and have no energy. I think back to the day before, and then remember indulging in pastries, ice cream and cake last night.

You must have had a bad reaction to one or all of these.

Example: I ate food at a restaurant and soon after, I start to feel sick at my stomach. Alternatively, I feel the beginnings of an adverse reaction to something.

In most cases, activated charcoal capsules and or strong hot tea can bring relief to mild food poisoning. If it is an extreme condition, it is important to obtain professional medical help as soon as possible. Remember charcoal will absorb out medications and may not be helpful in all cases. Charcoal can be bought over the counter to use at your own discretion, do further research for any question and see a doctor.

Example: My kidneys start to hurt more and more over several days. I think it must be due to something I am eating, drinking, or taking as a supplement.   Therefore, a negative affect is building up inside the kidneys.

The likely solution is to start an elimination-testing program to find the cause.

Example: I am diagnosed with multiple sclerosis (MS) or some other nervous system disorder. After some research, I understand the cause of this may be related to neurotoxins inside my body. Many food additives are neurotoxins or excitotoxins. Therefore, I begin the effort to remove any possible offending toxins.

Some possibilities are chelating treatments and fasting, along with cleaning up the diet and environment.

Example: I am a little overweight, out of shape and not happy. I decide I need a change. However, change is very difficult. Dieting is hard; also, my work and home life are stressful. I feel like I have little control over my life.

The first step is to study every resource that you can find, in health books, in spiritual information, and even on the internet looking for forums that are related to your specific situation. In addition, check out the local health food stores for products, and see if there are any helpful people. Also, check out the local gyms, churches and activity clubs. Formulate a plan to change lifestyle in a slow transitional manner in steps, by achieving little goals. Happiness is mostly a daily positive habit. A happy lifestyle does not depend on being wealthy.

Example: I am extremely overweight and most members of my family are overweight. Even with constant dieting, I am unable to get off the weight. Most people in my family are sickly and tend toward diabetes, heart disease and other chronic illnesses. Following Biblical Daniel's example, I am determined to better myself. I decide to avoid all manmade sugars, refined grains and most course grains. I eliminate all manmade processed foods except for rare treats. I eat mostly pulse foods in fresh, frozen, canned, dried, sprouted and fermented forms. I start an exercise and lifestyle improvement program. I give up all breads, cakes and cookies, even the homemade versions. I eat very little processed grains of any kind. I eat very little to zero dairy products. I add healthy oil into my foods, as I need, and a tiny bit of salt. To be exactly like Biblical Daniel is to eat no meat. However, if I do eat meat-I have tiny amounts and buy meat that is grass fed with no hormones or antibiotics. If I eat fish, it is clean wild caught fish.

You must be patient with yourself; a lifetime of bad habits is not easy to change. A body sick and overweight for many years cannot be made thin and strong in a few months. Since it took years to be in a bad condition it may take a few years to create the healthy thin body you want. Concentrate on making better lifestyle and diet rather than counting pounds the first few months to a year of effort. The first step toward better lifestyle may be working on self-esteem, by studying resources about this subject and finding support groups.

Example: *I am having itchy skin the last few weeks at odd places on my body, possibilities are* *on the belly, arms, and chest, or somewhere else.*

An itchy spot or rash anywhere on the body that will not go away is a sign of an adverse reaction to something. Many possible allergens will cause itchy skin, let us assume it is a nut or seed allergy. In this case, choose only one or two nuts to eat for a couple of weeks and see how your body responds. Keep on testing by adding or taking away, a nut or seed every two weeks until you find what you are allergic too. It is important not to over eat nuts and seeds because it is more likely to gain an allergy to them.

Example: *I am having nosebleeds lately and do not know why.*

Nosebleeds are an indication of high blood pressure created by an adverse reaction to something. Think about what you were eating or drinking right before the nose bleed. (We are assuming the nosebleeds are due to an adverse reaction to something)

Example: *Most people develop health problems as they age, name any pain, or ill health condition, this is their average approach to a cure. They go to a doctor and they demand a diagnosis-a name for their pain, and they demand a corresponding treatment. The doctor is always under this diagnosis-treatment "gun", every day, day after day, for patient after patient. The harried doctor is always short on time... The symptoms are discussed and tests are run. What is the result much of the time?   A possible* *disease is named with a mysterious or incurable cause. Pills are given to treat the symptoms, the patient is somewhat happy; they now have a name for their pain, and pills to take for it. The doctor is happy because the patient usually shuts up for awhile, and happiest of all is the pharmaceutical company who makes a profit. This dynamic repeats onward until the patient is taking 10 to 20 or more pills a day. It seems the upper limit of pills for a human body to take in a day is around 20 before it cannot take anymore... Of course, the patient is in a downward death spiral...*

I cannot tell you what to do, but I can tell you I think differently and act differently than most people. If I feel ill, I assume there is a real cause with a real cure. I think about what I am ingesting or breathing that is causing an ill effect. I think about adverse reactions from something in my environment, to identify and eliminate them. I *must* assume (right or wrong) that if I do the right thing I will get better and recover. The hardest part is in knowing what to do.

If chronically sick, I would start a relentless effort in research and experimentation to try to cure myself. If I were unable to make progress, I would certainly use professional help, choosing medical care professionals suitable to my approach.

Of course, I would take anything that is helpful for my health condition. However, my mindset for treating symptoms is the last resort, not the first choice. I would use whatever I had to for the moment, while searching for a real cure.

A simple example is artery clogging and high blood pressure. The real cure is changing diet in order to get the crud out of the arteries before a heart attack. I think most illnesses have a simple cure, if only people knew what to do and have the fortitude to do it.

Be careful of taking anything that is manmade or unnaturally concentrated by man from natural sources for too long. Consider elimination testing anything your ingesting of this nature.

Most sicknesses are because of something adverse put into the mouth or a lack of something in the diet. Some illnesses are because of something toxic breathed in or absorbed into the skin. The afflicted person can solve these kinds of health problems in most cases with study and effort.

Chapter Twenty One

Ten-day challenges

If a person is sickly or grossly overweight, it is best to check with a health care provider to discuss exercise.

Here is a lifestyle challenge. During the next ten days, obtain a new hobby, something that encourages you to be in better shape and to exercise. Here is a list of physically active hobbies to consider.

Hiking, mountaineering, jogging, paintball, mountain biking, road biking, walking, caving, basketball, golf, martial arts, swimming, back country fishing, wild plant gathering, and orienteering. Find competitions, such as iron man or iron woman contests, 10K races and marathon runs, or planning for fun trips, such as hiking trips or mountaineering trips. Think about how to gain new skills while exercising, such as participating in martial arts. Exercise can be part of a positive daily lifestyle, such as riding to work on a bicycle.

It is possible to do adventure trips, or to join a local outdoor activity group such as the scouts. You can join a rescue group, or become a volunteer firefighter. You will need to be in physical shape for these hobbies and will have new interesting skills to learn.

Choose at least one new hobby that encourages you to be in physical condition. The best kinds are those that motivate you to train. If you already have a physical hobby, is it fresh enough to motivate you?   Think about new variations to try or even a new hobby.

Another kind of challenge is a diet challenge. A cleansing ten-day challenge is simple, eat no meat and have only clean pulse foods for ten days. This means eating only seeds, nuts, fruits, vegetables, and grains. Eat very little processed breads, and buy the simplest natural breads. They are in local bakeries. Simple meal choices can be beans with rice or vegetables with rice or oatmeal with nuts. Have salads with beans and cottage cheese. Dairy is a common allergen that many should avoid except maybe a little cottage cheese, organic butter and yogurt. How you feel when eating any dairy product is the final guide.

The only beverages allowed are water, fruit juices and a little herbal tea. I suggest on average no more than two glasses of fruit juice a day. No more than one cup of herbal tea a day and the rest is water.

Here is a starter list of foods to avoid or limit, cheese, milk, non-organic corn products, non-organic foods, commercial breads. No roasted nuts, eat only raw nuts and seeds, no high sugar content products. Avoid processed food products, coffee, regular teas with caffeine and alcohol. Eat little to zero meat and chocolate of any kind. Avoid or limit exotic to you foods and beverages. Eat pulse kinds of foods, to make them tasty, use healthy oil, salt, and a few natural condiments.

Ingest little or no processed wheat based

products such as common white wheat pasta.

If you have arthritis, consider giving up the nightshade family of vegetables during your ten-day period as a test. These are tomatoes, peppers, eggplant and potatoes. Sweet potatoes are fine to eat and are healthy.

I suggest eating as much food as you desire during your initial transition toward better health. This means no restrictions for food eaten because it will be hard enough to change the kinds of food you eat. After ten days of cleaner diet, you should be able to tell the foods you have an adverse reaction too. Then, you can bring foods and beverages back one at a time and see how your body reacts.

Another challenge for ten days is to start a new exercise program, if out of shape start slowly. I suggest walking and easy resistance training. Walking on a flat surface gives very little exercise unless speed walking, but is fine when starting out. Walk for at least thirty minutes a day and go as long as forty-five minutes to an hour. Work up to hill walking and use a light backpack for greater challenge when needed.

I suggest alternating workouts, for instance for those days not walking get in a resistance exercise program. I prefer weight training in a gym, or doing push-ups, sit-ups and chin-ups at home. Do not miss a chance to push mow a lawn or to do some moderate outdoor physical work. Try to get in three workouts a week, along with an active weekend.

Few things are as brutal for an evening person than a morning workout. Nevertheless, if you have the desire to lose weight and keep it off as a permanent lifestyle, then consider doing all your workouts first thing in the morning before breakfast. This will set the body's metabolism to be higher and I find that my desire to eat bad foods is less during the day. It is also helpful to spend a few minutes before you get out of bed to think about yourself, God, and the coming day; this is a kind of daily meditation. As a ten-day challenge consider doing all your workouts in the morning and see how it works for you.

My suggestions may not work perfectly for everyone, experiment to find your own way in daily exercise. For instance, my wife likes yard work and mowing the grass, but she does not enjoy formal exercise.

Unfortunately, eating out is usually not that healthy. Many people eat out daily for convenience and companionship, but it may not be a good idea for health. Balance social needs with the need for good clean food. Once again, the wife and I were hungry and running late so we stopped at a local Chinese restaurant with a great buffet for our second meal. Many good foods were there, we ate fruit, grains, vegetables and no meat, and had a great time with very tasty food. Nevertheless, the next day we both felt hung over.

Everyday when you wake up judge how you feel. When healthy you should feel good in the morning, with energy, if not usually something is wrong. This morning we both felt hung over, so something was wrong with the food last night. I do not know exactly what, but I suspect the oil or an additive (MSG). At home, we use clean olive oil for most cooking, and most restaurants use cheaper oil. Cheap oils are often genetically modified and made with unhealthy processing. The source foods in restaurants may be healthy, but it is difficult to avoid the cheaper oils and additives. Use how you feel as a guide when choosing restaurants.

If you eat out at restaurants and most of us do, here is a ten-day challenge. For ten days eat only healthy home-prepared foods and raw foods, and be strict. See how you feel especially in the morning, and then afterward eat only restaurant foods for several days in a row. Choose your normal favorite restaurants, see how you feel and compare.

Ten-day two meals a day dieting challenges

Why should you complete a two meals a day diet challenge? It will test your resolve to eat only two meals a day for ten days without further commitment.

If you desire and need to lose weight consult with your medical care provider. A way to lose weight and keep it off is to eat two meals a day with little to zero snacking. To eat two meals a day takes desire and willpower. However, after ten days, you will find it easier, I promise. Your mind and body will start to adapt to this program.

In order to lose weight the natural way a person must burn more calories than taken in. It is a common mistake to diet and restrict calories without exercise. It is better to restrict calories a little with enough nutrition to have a workout program.   There are many different ways to diet and some programs claim to have a way to lose weight without feeling hungry. I think this is clever marketing, but not realistic. At least until your body adapts to a better lifestyle.

Why are two meals a day a positive lifestyle option? Two reasons, one, it gives your digestive organs and body time to rest in between meals. Therefore, the digestive organs can process out food before the next meal is stacked on top. When the second meal is finished before 6pm, the food is out of the stomach sooner. This enables the body to focus on healing at night rather than endlessly digesting. The second reason is that with only two meals a day you can eat until full at mealtime without counting calories. Eating healthy balanced meals, you will have the right amount of food with only two meals a day. You can snack on this program, but if the snacks become meals then you are off the program. Snacks should be low calorie simple foods such as raw fruit, raw vegetables, a bit of raw nuts and seeds. The stricter you are with two meals a day with little snacking, the more weight you will lose.

In between the morning meal and the second evening meal, you can have a piece of fruit for lunch if you need, any food easy to digest. The more sedentary you are the better the two meals a day works. It is more difficult to overeat on two meals a day. If you need to snack more than with one piece of fruit during the mid-day, do so with more fruit, raw vegetables and a small amount of raw nuts and seeds. This is the best way to stay on the program. Raw snack foods are healthy, easy to digest and have fewer calories. If you eat or drink processed foods as snacks, you are off the diet.

To start the day, the first thing in the morning squeeze one fresh lemon, put the juice in a quart of warm water, drink this as the morning drink. It flushes and cleans the kidneys. Around fifteen minutes after this lemon drink have a full nutritious breakfast; eat until full, do not count calories (Assuming you are eating healthy foods).

For mid-day pack raw foods for light snacking, you may take only a single food item to be strict. Such as a single apple, you may add in a handful of nuts and seeds for fat and protein. The evening meal is the same, make a balanced nutritious meal and eat until full. That is all the food for the day.

I would be cautious about a two meals a day diet challenge for children, pregnant women or younger teenagers. If children have a weight problem, it is likely due to eating too much processed fatty and carbohydrate-laden foods along with a low amount of activity. Children need to eat more often than two meals a day because they have small stomachs. I do not recommend a strict two meals a day for children. See a health care professional for overweight children. Use good sense for children's diets, because they need nutrition while growing.

This is a typical two meals a day schedule. Eat a full breakfast, hot oatmeal with raw nuts and fruit. Go to work, for lunch have raw fruits and vegetables, a small amount of nuts and a little more of raw seeds. I personally like pumpkin seeds the best. They are very healthy. Then have a home cooked second meal, an example is rice, beans, salad, and vegetables. This is the daily two meals program, which can be done as a ten-day challenge.

If you are overweight and cannot get the fat off, a strict two meals program should do it when eating pulse foods and exercising. You will feel some hunger in between meals and during late evening; this is as it should be. The weight will come off very slow, which is correct in a lifestyle that you can keep up. However, if you are still having problems losing weight, then reduce the mid day snacks as much as needed, all the way to zero and increase healthy exercise. In addition, you may reduce fat and oil intake.

A more strenuous ten-day challenge for dieting is to eat a raw foods meal for one of the two meals. For instance, eat a salad with olive oil and vinegar or lemon juice as the dressing; eat any kind of raw fruit or vegetable or nuts and seeds. The calories for raw foods are low, so eat until full, the weight will still come off. A strenuous ten-day challenge is no mid-day snacking and eating one of the two meals as a raw foods only meal.

In my personal experience with eating two meals a day, it is difficult at first, then the mind and body adapts. This adaptation takes about ten days to a month. As a ten-day challenge stick to eating two meals with zero or very light snacking. To lose weight it is best to have no mid-day snacking or just one piece of fruit.

After ten days (if you make it) keep on going until you are at a reasonable target weight. Let us say your target weight is 180 pounds, be on a strict two meals a diet until about 178 pounds. Then you may start eating raw foods for mid-day snacking while watching weight. If weight goes up above the target, then back to two strict meals a day until back to target weight.

It is best to have a daily schedule, to *check weight every day*, like after the morning shower. If you want to maintain weight by this program be strict about checking weight as a daily habit.

Variations

1. Ten days of two meals a day with unlimited raw foods snacking during mid-day: (This is ineffective for losing weight for most, people unless working hard, but it should prevent weight gain when active.)

2. Ten days of two meals a day with unlimited snacking midday while eating very low calorie natural foods. (This is for those people who need to fill themselves up midday. Strictly limit all higher calorie natural foods such as olives, avocados, dried fruit, nuts and seeds. Eat lots of fresh or lightly cooked vegetables and fruits prepared in a plain simple way.)

3. Ten days of two meals a day with a single piece of fruit mid-day with a small handful of raw nuts and seeds: (It is more

effective when eating only a single piece of fruit and nothing else).

4. Ten days of two meals a day with zero mid-day snacking.

5. Ten days of two meals a day, the morning meal made up of raw fruits, vegetables, nuts, seeds or lightly cooked fruits and vegetables, no fats, grains or meat. You can moderately snack midday with raw foods but eating very few nuts, dried fruits or any other high calorie natural foods. The key here is no grains, fats, sugars, meats, white potatoes (i.e., no higher calorie natural foods) for breakfast and snacking. In the evening have a full meal with whatever healthy food you desire, including the higher calorie natural foods such as rice, potatoes and grains.

6. Ten days of two meals a day, one meal is a raw foods meal with the healthiest juices and zero snacking.

7. Ten days of eating two meals a day, no snacking, and a juice fast one day out of ten days. (After the ten days, juice fast one day a week until you meet target weight. A juice fast is drinking only juice for food the whole day)

In all ten-day diet challenges, if you desire, keep on going after the ten days until your target weight is met, then monitor. If you are not losing weight, then go on a stricter program. If you are losing too much weight or feeling weak, then go on a less strict program. Any of these programs can be a permanent lifestyle change, experiment and find what works for you. Other variations are possible as long as they are healthy.

When losing fat weight it should be about a pound or less a week, same for gaining weight, about a pound or less a week. It is possible to gain and lose water weight at greater rate. You need to know the difference-if you are thirsty and weight is lower, then you lost water weight. If you are full of water and heavier, this means a gain in water weight. Be sure if you are on a strict two meals a day to eat some raw foods at the two meals.

This is a slow program of weight loss. It may take a few months to notice a weight change, especially in the winter. It is easier to lose weight in summer because of more activity.

You may tend to overeat at the two meals until you get used to the program. If you over eat at the two meals, slowly transition so you eat until full, but not bloated. If you feel hungry before the next mealtime (without going to an extreme), you are eating the right amount. Another effective dieting method is to reduce fat and oil in meals while still getting enough.

If you are having trouble losing weight, eat only pulse foods to get the weight off and keep it off. That means no manmade high glycemic index foods, no sugars, excessive fats or refined flours. Even homemade cookies, cakes or breads have fats, refined flours and sugars in them, so should be avoided. The stricter you are the easier weight control will be.

If you want natural treats, then plan them into meals as a dessert. Two meals a day can be

a   permanent   lifestyle.   It   can   maintain   a
healthy weight for the rest of your life.

Chapter Twenty Two

Vitamins and minerals

It is difficult to eat enough in order to obtain all the nutrients that your body can use. Especially when eating today's modern processed food. It is too easy to eat pasta or bread products or other easy to prepare products that do not have enough nutrition. Even people who are trying to eat healthier often do not get enough nutrients. It is possible to get enough nutrients by only eating food, but it takes an extra effort to avoid processed foods and to eat healthy.

How many people eat large helpings of greens every week? Not many I would estimate. What about you, did you have greens today? I sometimes buy a green health drink from the health food store or I make fresh juice, this helps. I suggest buying and or growing organic food as much as you can. I also suggest only taking food based vitamins and minerals as a complex, if you take a vitamin supplement. Why food based? There are two schools of thought and I have my own experience. I have heard that chemically made vitamins are as effective and safe as vitamins made naturally in plants or animals. I also heard that chemically made vitamins are artificial and harsh on the body.

Nutrients processed inside plants have a different origin. The plant brings nutrients up from the roots and incorporates these into it, or manufactures the nutrients. If you think about it, plants are the natural source to get nutrients. Ancient people did not grind up rocks to get their vitamins and minerals. They did gather some salt if they could, that is about all. The best for health is sea salt but commercial table salt has added iodine, which is good because iodine is a common deficiency. Consider using sea salt with added iodine.

I believe for long-term health and gentleness on organs, it is best to use food based vitamins and minerals as much as possible. A further step up in health may to obtain all needed nutrition from food and not risk unknown organ damage due to long-term supplementation. Vitamins and minerals in food is part of a complex inside the food, it is not a group of pure chemicals, which may be harsh on the system. Whether to use supplementation or not, is a choice that each individual must make for themselves and if so what kind and how long. I myself lean toward using little supplementation, mainly because of my sensitive kidneys and wanting to avoid the risk of unforeseen damage.

In my hierarchy of supplementation, the least desirable are the chemically made kinds, second least are those that are food based with processing, and the best are the least processed 100% food based supplements. Note, even natural herbal supplements can have harsh effects in the body and organs for some individuals. Use how you feel as your main guide, so pay attention to how your organs feel on any supplement program.

I have sensitive kidneys, and these are my

detectors of harsh supplements. If I have kidney pain, I cannot take the supplement. Unlike most people, I can usually tell the difference between harsh and gentle supplements. I sometimes can take a brand of supplements that are 100% whole food supplements. These are food based and unlike most supplements, they can be taken by themselves on an empty stomach.

There is a disadvantage in real food supplementation. The concentration in each pill is much lower than the chemically made supplements. Nevertheless, the advantage is that supplementation from food-based products is less likely to harm organs.

Kidney failure is becoming more common these days. I suspect that this is because of poor choices in beverages and foods by people. In addition, this can be a trend for those trying to be healthier by taking harsh supplements for too long. For the last year, I have been taking no supplements at all and have good health. You do not need supplements to be healthy; you do need good diet and lifestyle.

Beware of what you are ingesting, because even some of the items from a health food store may be harsh on your organs. I got my sensitive kidneys primarily from drinking too much green tea. I cannot get them to recover back 100% to what they were originally. They are compromised and weaker than they should due to my mistake. I understood green tea to be a healthy drink so I drank about a quart of strong jasmine green tea a day for a few years. That was a mistake.

I later on learned for some people excessive tea drinking causes crystals to form in the kidneys. Also too much protein, especially protein from supplements can be hard on the kidneys. I also took some vitamin powders that may have been harsh on my organs. At the time, I did not know to be careful of my kidneys with such drinks and supplements. Watch out for this effect.

People who train to be stronger may take protein supplements, if you are doing so, be careful and not overdo it. I think it better for long-term health not to take protein supplementation, at least be aware and moderate the intake.

I must say I think my kidneys are my weakest point in my organ health today and regret their injury. This happened due to a lack of knowledge and information for me at that time. It is important for us to read every good health information source we can find. Study information from many expert sources and cross check. It is important to watch how you feel and stop any new practice the instant you feel an adverse effect.

It is known that soils can be deficient in certain vital nutrients and this can cause deficiencies. At my current residence in Washington State, selenium and zinc concentrations are low in the soil. In today's modern world, we get food shipped to everywhere, but still this is good to know.

I do not favor taking large amounts of any single vitamin or mineral for long periods of time. I think this can cause imbalances in the body, and create an ill effect. I favor taking gentle balanced formulas of vitamins and minerals, if I take anything at all. The only current exception to that rule is that I take vitamin D in the winter.

I sometimes have cramps in my legs and toes. In the past, I took a natural food based formula made up of magnesium calcium and potassium with some additional salt.   It is common for potassium, calcium and magnesium to be deficient in the body, which creates health problems. Another way is to increase intake of greens and raw nuts and seeds, I have done this in recent times with good effect. It is possible to take a certain supplement and cause health problems, as too much of one mineral or vitamin can cause imbalances.

I personally find that it is difficult to figure out what my body needs in terms of minerals and vitamins by only how I feel. The safest long-term practice in supplementation is using a balanced formula in the least harsh form you can find. I think the best chance for a long healthy lifespan is to obtain nutrition from raw and lightly cooked fresh organic foods.

Years ago, I used to take a high dosage of vitamin C, but I did not balance it out with added calcium and other minerals. This was a mistake since high doses of C leach out calcium; once again, this was due to a lack of information. The expert I followed did not mention this possible problem. In addition, there are no warning labels about this on vitamin C containers. I am much healthier today because of my active involvement in health. Nevertheless, I made some mistakes along the way, every mistake due to a lack of information.

Personally, I am cautious of any new wonderful supplement on the market. Science studies and personal experiences may be great and true. Nevertheless, short-term science studies and personal experiences may not indicate harmful effects long term. Most everything, which has strong effect, will have side effects that vary from person to person. If you take any kind of supplementation or pills, anything at all watch how you feel carefully.

Chapter Twenty Three

List of common deficiencies

Iron: About 2% of men and 5% of women are deficient in the USA; it is the most common deficiency in the world. Symptoms are weakness, pinkish blood rather than red blood, pale skin, hair loss, shortness of breath. Iron is important for endurance. Women lose Iron due to pregnancy and menstrual cycles. The common source of iron is red meat, and there are many plant and nut sources of iron. However if you are a vegetarian, there is a greater chance of being deficient. There is evidence that additional iron may increase endurance for work and exercise even when not noticeably deficient. Consider iron supplementation if you do not eat meat, or for pregnant women, athletes and people who do hard physical work.

The recommended daily amount of iron is about 10mg for men and 20mg for women. 1/4 cup raw sunflower seeds = 2.6mg; 1/4 cup raisins = 1.3mg; 1/4 cup pumpkin seeds = 8.5 mg; 1/4 cup raw almonds = 2mg; 1 cup cooked lentils = 6.6 mg; 1 cup cooked spinach = 6mg.

Calcium: It is used throughout the body and in the bones and teeth. Symptoms of deficiency are muscle cramping, soft weak teeth with many cavities, weak bones, dry skin and brittle fingernails. If you take a lot of vitamin C without additional calcium, deficiency may develop. In addition, a person sweats out calcium when working and may need additional calcium. You need magnesium in balance with calcium, two parts calcium to one part magnesium. It is possible to be slightly deficient in calcium with no obvious symptoms and this will erode health.

Ancient man had plenty of calcium without dairy, from tubers, greens, insects and bones. While today, many people are deficient. Modern people can also obtain calcium from bones by using soup bones and eating fish with the bones cooked inside the meat. Bone has a two to one ratio of calcium to phosphorous, rather than just calcium alone. Modern day possibilities for more calcium are canned salmon and sardines, both are high in bone content. I used to eat canned salmon, but I would often get sick. I do not know if it is an allergy or due to tainted meat, most likely an allergy. I never have a problem with canned sardines. There are herbal-based supplements for calcium, but these are low in concentration.

In today's modern world, some experts assume that people will eat dairy products for calcium. For people who avoid dairy, it can be difficult to obtain the daily USA calcium recommendation of around 1000mg without supplementation. Consider supplementation if you do not eat dairy. However, some people think that 300 to 500mg of calcium a day is enough because most of world ingests this amount daily. In addition, the world health organization indicates 500mg of calcium a day is enough. It is easy to obtain 300 to 500mg of calcium a day when eating healthy pulse foods. Being low in vitamin D causes much less uptake of calcium. Having enough vitamin D is important to make use of the calcium you do eat.

The recommendation is to have 500 to 1200 mg of calcium a day. 4 ounces canned sardines = 500mg; 4 ounces canned salmon = 360mg; (Four ounces of meat is about half the palm of your hand) 1/2 cup or four ounces of tofu = 145mg; 1 tablespoon of blackstrap molasses = 137mg; 1/2 cup of cottage cheese = 100mg; 1/4 cup raw almonds= 95mg; 1 tablespoon of sesame seeds = 90mg; 1/2 cup of cooked kale = 103mg; 1 tablespoon of raw chia seeds = 123mg; 1 cup of yogurt = 450mg; 1 cup of broccoli = 178mg; 10 figs = 270mg.

Vitamin D: Deficiency is because of lack of sunlight and seafood. Deficiency can cause mild depression, weak bones, soft teeth, and many other illness symptoms. During the winter months, you may take vitamin D for better mood and energy. Supplementation is more important for northern people to keep a good mood. Enough vitamin D is very important for the absorption of calcium. You may use sun lamps for naturally created vitamin D. Some foods high in vitamin D are mackerel, salmon, herring, sardines, tuna fish, cod liver oil (most fish have vitamin D) and eggs. In the winter months, you need to eat plenty of fish and or supplement with vitamin D. I take a vitamin D supplement in the wintertime; this greatly helps my mood and energy. I do eat plenty of organic eggs, but I feel I need more vitamin D. Nuts and seeds have no vitamin D.

It is recommended to have 600IU of vitamin D a day. One can of sardines = 516IU. All fish are high in vitamin D. It is good to get around thirty minutes of sunlight two to three times a week. I live in a northern area so I like to sit in my car in the sunshine during winter. You can warm the car with its heater and take a nap with some exposed skin. Alternatively, if a house window is orientated correctly you can do this in the home.

Chromium: Chromium supplementation may help people with diabetes, but if you have diabetes consult your physician to make sure there isn't interference with medications. Deficiency in chromium is considered somewhat rare. Signs are low blood sugar and mood swings. A diet high in refined sugar will lower chromium levels in the body. Foods high in chromium are nutritional yeast, brewer's yeast, (nutritional yeast has good flavor, brewers yeast does not), fruits and vegetables, meats and whole grains.

Magnesium: A symptom of deficiency is muscle cramping. Magnesium works to let muscles relax after contraction. A diet sufficient in magnesium helps to prevent heart attack and will lower blood pressure. Deficiency of magnesium may cause mental problems such as anxiety, depression, forgetfulness and fatigue. An elevated dose for a short period may help someone recover from mental problems such as depression or manic-depressive mood swings. Then drop down to a suggested daily dosage, see a physician for this possible treatment. Research indicates most people are deficient in magnesium. If a person eats junk foods and drinks, such as soda, coffee and alcohol then they are likely to be deficient. In addition, calcium supplementation without magnesium can cause deficiency in magnesium. Some foods high in magnesium are rice bran, wheat bran, oat bran, squash seeds, pumpkin seeds, watermelon seeds, sesame seeds, sunflower seeds, and almonds. I personally had muscle cramps for many years and the best solution for me is eating little salt, raw nuts, seeds and organic greens. I try to eat 2-4 handfuls of pumpkin seeds every day. I tried magnesium and mineral supplements with only partial improvement.

It is recommended to have 300 to 450 mg of magnesium a day: 1/4 cup of raw pumpkin seeds = 185mg: 1/2 cup rice bran = 460mg: 1/2 cup wheat bran = 180mg: 1/2 cup oat bran = 110mg: 1/4 cup raw almonds = 96 mg: 1/4 cup raw cashews = 94 mg: 1 avocado = 112 mg: 1/4 cup raw sunflower seeds = 114mg: 1/4 cup molasses = 204mg: 1 banana = 58mg: 1 cup oatmeal = 50mg: 1 cup kale = 23mg: 1 cup brown rice = 84mg.

In general, if you eat 1/4 cup to a cup of mixed raw nuts and seeds along with good non-processed foods you are likely getting enough magnesium. If you eat mostly processed foods, you are not getting enough magnesium. If your drinking water is high in magnesium, you can get away with less magnesium in your diet.

Potassium: A main symptom of deficiency is muscle cramping, also excessive thirst and frequent urination. Some foods high in potassium are apricots, figs, dates, peaches, raisins, bananas, yogurt, avocados, and greens (kale, spinach, etc). In today's world of processed foods and cooking, potassium levels are too low and salt levels are too high. Cooking destroys potassium. Processed foods are low in potassium. Canned foods are low in potassium. Man in ancient times could not get much salt, but got plenty of potassium. Potassium levels are high in the raw natural foods that ancient man ate. The body is designed to hold salt and to get rid of potassium. Many people are chronically low in potassium and too high in salt due to the modern diet.

Ancient man ingested around one to three grams of salt a day on average from his foods. In a level teaspoon there is about 6 grams of salt. (Note, six grams of salt taken all at once may kill a person). Other than potassium supplementation, it is better to eat raw and lightly cooked foods and have moderate salt intake, especially if you have kidney and or high blood pressure problems. On a two meals a day program, eat meals with plenty of raw foods and eat snacks exclusively made up of raw foods.

The need for potassium per day is around 2000 milligrams a day, more if exercising hard. The highest sources of potassium in common foods are one banana=440 mg; 1 cup, raisins =

1100 mg; 1 cup, orange juice = 496mg; 1 avocado = 1400mg; 1 potato = 782mg; 1 fish, 4 ounces (Which is about half the palm of your hand) = 550mg.

Sea Salt: Most people eat plenty of salt, so it is not a common deficiency. However, if you go on a health diet do not make the mistake of restricting salt too much, especially if you are exercising and sweating a lot. Signs of deficiency are muscle cramping such as foot and leg cramping. Some commercially made salts have iodine in them and sea salt normally does not. Consider buying sea salt with added iodine. Salt with iodine typically has the bare minimum amount of iodine, not the optimum amount. It is somewhat common for people to go on a health diet and not get enough salt. Alternatively, excess salt intake raises blood pressure and is hard on the kidneys. Ancient man ingested about 1/6 to 1/2 level teaspoons of salt a day out of their foods. Ancient man typically did not add salt in food; his salt came from food. Therefore, the body is designed to be very efficient in keeping and using salt. As a rule of thumb, do not add more than 1/2 a level teaspoon of salt into your cooked food a day, per person. A level teaspoon of salt is 6 grams. The optimum amount of salt to add into prepared food can be less, maybe about 1/4 a level teaspoon a day, unless sweating a lot. Much depends on how you eat; if you eat processed foods, these are often high in salt. If you decide to lower salt intake, give your body time to adjust and make sure you are getting all other needed minerals.

A very rough guide for salt use is to add into the food you cook about 1/6 to 1/3 teaspoon of salt a day-if you eat some processed foods with salt. If you eat many processed foods containing salt, then do not add salt to your food. If you eat zero processed salty foods, add about half a teaspoon (3 grams) a day--plus or minus a forth of a teaspoon. As always, use how you feel as a primary guide to raise and lower salt intake. It is better if you are muscle cramping to increase first *calcium, magnesium, and potassium* from natural food sources and see how you feel. Avoid loading up on salt as a first option. Most people are more likely to be too high in salt intake than too low. Eat less salt if you have kidney pain, high blood pressure and heart trouble.

Note: several combinations of deficiency or excess in minerals and vitamins can cause muscle cramping and other health problems. Short term it may be beneficial to do a single mineral supplementation in excess if needed. Long-term minerals must be in balance inside the body or health problems can develop.

Iodine: Deficiency affects about 40% of the world's population. This can cause many health problems, such as thyroid enlargement, and mental retardation for children of deficient mothers. Salt with iodine has the minimum needed to prevent goiter, not necessarily the optimum amount for health. Some foods high in iodine are seaweed, cod, tuna, and eggs. Consider iodine supplementation and eat plenty of seaweed, kelp, and fish.

Vitamin B and B12: Lack of B vitamins is a common deficiency. Deficiency symptoms are impaired mental function, numbness and tingling of skin, a feeling of pins and needles, and anemia. Vitamin B is important for maximum mental function for students. I eat nutritional yeast regularly to get plenty of B vitamins. It is very tasty in foods. Other sources are greens, almonds, pecans, fish, meats, and grains.

Trace minerals: A lack of molybdenum, selenium, phosphorus, iodine, potassium, sodium, zinc and others will cause many health problems. If you are deficient in one of these, it is likely you are deficient in others. If so, you can take a balanced mineral formula. You may want to increase intake for a week or two and then lower down to a suggested daily dosage. For long-term health, the best habit is to eat plenty of organic vegetables, fruits, seeds and nuts.

You should aim to get needed nutrition by eating plenty of organic raw fruits, vegetables, dried fruits, sprouted seeds, nuts and seeds and so on. Organic foods should be naturally fertilized and non-GMO. This means organic farmers add into the soil organic mulch and manure, making the soil rich in all nutrients. These nutrients are incorporated into the plant as it grows. If the soil is not organically fertilized enough it can become exhausted and low in nutrition. Thus, the plants are lower in nutrition. *Most farm soil is low in nutrition as compared to fresh soil, due to hundreds of years of usage.*

As a practical manner to afford food, many people eat non-organic foods and risk not getting enough nutrition. They can make it up by supplementation, but risk unknown damage by many years of supplementation. It is better to grow a small greens garden and spend extra money on natural and organic foods. Some natural foods that you prepare from scratch are cheaper than processed foods.

Nutritional deficiency in developing babies and children can cause problems that could last for a lifetime. Women trying to get pregnant should take a multiple vitamin mineral supplement for some time before pregnancy and during pregnancy. There are many stories about pregnant women losing health such as tooth/bone strength (calcium loss) due to the baby's development.

If you have muscle cramping, consider mineral supplements in a balanced formula. Likely, if you are deficient enough to have cramping, you need minerals and vitamins in a balanced whole foods formula and maybe a little extra salt. Other problems and diseases can cause cramping as well, see a doctor as needed. For instance too much of a single mineral may cause cramping, too much salt will leach calcium out of the body, etc.

If you are exercising hard, sweating and processing more than an average amount of liquids and foods; the need for vitamins and minerals may increase over the recommended daily amount. When deficient you are not at your true potential. However, be careful not to overdo any single supplement and get the body out of balance. I personally find the safest practice is a balanced broad-spectrum vitamin supplement, but you may need extra potassium, calcium, and magnesium. The absolute best is getting all nutrition by eating the right kinds of foods, with very little supplementation.

Coffee, tea, soda, distilled water or any beverage of this sort in excess can create a diuretic effect. This means when you drink the beverage its liquid goes into balance with the mineral filled liquid in your body, then you pee it out. The net effect is to remove minerals and nutrients out of the body. A person can become deficient over a long period of time, usually it takes months to years. This will erode health, so limit diuretic beverages. Eat plenty of nutritious food, and take balanced mineral/vitamin supplements when needed.

My personal experience lately: I daily eat a few handfuls of raw seeds and nuts. I try to eat 1/4 of a cup, to a 3/4 cup of a mixture of raw nuts and seeds. Every day I try to eat fresh fruit, raw vegetables and dried fruit. This is a big nutritional help for me along with eating cooked greens, such as kale, around two times a week. I make a big bowl of greens seasoned with healthy oil, a little salt and a tablespoon of apple cider vinegar. (Note; white vinegar is not very healthy. Apple cider vinegar is very healthy.)

To be similar to Biblical Daniel does not mean exercising hard and eating processed foods with treats, then as an afterthought eat some healthy foods. It means a huge effort to eat correctly with zero bad foods and having a positive lifestyle with moderate exercise. If you do this, you will have health, endurance, strength and a clear mind into old age.

As you get older, especially past the mid thirties, small unhealthy treats even on a weekly basis will erode health greater than in youth. It is best to eliminate such bad habits. For example, I recently drank a store bought peppermint hot chocolate and suffered a headache all afternoon. Even if you do not feel an acute ill effect from it, something bad eaten daily can erode health.

Chapter Twenty Four
Water

As I mentioned earlier, several years ago, I used to drink distilled water and no other water; I did so for about three years. This caused me to be anemic in iron and other nutrients. Unfortunately, distilled water is a diuretic, and will cause a loss of nutrients out of urine over time. If you drink distilled water over a long time, you must take in enough extra minerals and vitamins to replace what you lose.

Why does this happen? Distilled water is pure H2O with no minerals, so the minerals inside your body have to come into equilibrium with it. Then when you pee, you remove some of the body's minerals and nutrients. Normal spring or well water has minerals dissolved into solution with the water. Over a long period, months to years, distilled water will likely harm health. I think drinking distilled water may be fine to help in cleansing-for a few days to a few weeks, and may be fine long term with additional supplementation.

Any kind of diuretic beverage or medicine may have an anemic effect over a long time by removing nutrients when you pee. A common example is excessively drinking tea, coffee and soda. This coupled with poor nutrition can lead to vitamin and mineral deficiencies. Possible signs are soft teeth (cavities), muscle cramping, and lack of bone strength, bad posture, joint problems and overall ill health.

I like clean well water the best, if you are lucky to have it. In today's world, a practical solution is using a filtration system of some kind, such as reverse osmosis or a charcoal filter. I have been using a charcoal filter on tap water with good results.

Normal water has minerals desolved in solution with pure water. If the mineral content is elevated with limestone, it may cause kidney stones, something to be aware of in some parts of the country. A possible solution is drinking distilled water, but this may be worse for health in the long term due to the diuretic effect. Other possible solutions are buying spring water for drinking or mixing distilled water with tap water, or drinking distilled water with supplementation.

I know of a boy who is chronically ill partly due to well water that had arsenic in it. It happened because of the fruit farms in the area using pesticides over many years. The contaminated surface water went into the well water. I suggest that everyone have his or her water tested and or putting on a filter system.

Chemicals in water can come from toxic surface run off, from farms, industrial usage, even from people's medications when they use the bathroom. Treated water from a town or city most often has chorine, which is necessary to kill bacteria. However, it is otherwise unhealthy. Public water may have fluoride in it as well; fluoride increases the uptake of lead into the body. Unless you are in a pristine area that is isolated, you likely need water filtration. It is a cheap insurance for health.

A common problem is people not drinking enough water and drinking other beverages instead of water when thirsty. For full health and lifespan it is important to drink plenty of water, some people do not feel thirsty for water as they should. Everyone should drink about two quarts of clean water a day.

For homework, go to the local hardware store and check out the water filters. There should be charcoal filters that you can use on your tap water. Look for inexpensive replacement filters so you can afford to replace them regularly. You can find options that are more expensive online, but if on a budget look in the local hardware stores. There are more expensive filtration options out there such as reverse osmosis. But an inexpensive charcoal filter works great.

Chapter Twenty-Five
Herbals and homeopathic treatments

I think strong herbs and homeopathies are good short term for acute symptoms and illnesses, but I would not take them long term. Most strong medicinal herbs should not be taken for more than a couple of weeks then cycle off them for a while and back on as needed. Be careful with medicinal herbs, they can be powerful and often have negative side effects. It can be acceptable to use low dosage medicinal herbs and homeopathies long term when their effect is mild. If you are experimenting, monitor closely how you feel. The best practice is to do research beforehand or risk suffering.

One can use culinary herbs or spices long term. These are milder in effect and are to flavor or scent a food. Examples are garlic, ginger, cayenne pepper, cinnamon cilantro, bay leaf, basil, curry, dill, oregano, pepper, rosemary, sage, sassafras, vanilla, and wintergreen.

In my personal experience with herbs, there are culinary herbs that you can eat in food or take in a regular basis, in reasonable amounts, such as garlic or cayenne pepper for health. Second, there is a medicinal class of herbs that are usually used short term, or cycle on and off depending on the herb and need.

When considering medicinal herbs such as the aloe plant for intestinal cleansing of parasites and healing, you need to be careful. Short-term usage is the safest practice and monitor carefully how you feel. The general rule is to take medicinal herbs short term for a purpose and be off them. Alternatively, cycle off and on if you need to, for instance two weeks on and two weeks off. Rarely should a person take a strong medicinal herb continuously long term, especially for years and decades. If you do so, it is best to do the mildest effective dosage.

I personally do not do well on some herbal treatments, like drinking store bought aloe juice long term or using fenugreek tea. I do not react well to these and get liver pains, so I do not use them. Some people report that they drink small amounts of Aloe Vera juice every day for years with good effect. It is best to monitor your own condition and let this be the judge for you.

Another example is using a mild dosage of Echinacea and Goldenseal for influenzas and colds. One may take them during the winter season for three months and then go off them for the rest of the year.

I once had toothpicks with Tea Tree Oil in them and they made my mouth sore and numb after a few weeks of usage. I used about four toothpicks a day, until I figured out this negative effect. Tea Tree Oil takes special care in usage. I know of a friend who rubbed Tea Tree Oil into his pet kittens to get rid of fleas, and it killed the kittens. It has a powerful damaging effect on the nervous system. You can feel a numbing effect with its usage on the skin.

Remember, just because something is

natural, and you can buy it at a health store, it does not mean you do not have to be knowledgeable and careful in its usage. In some countries (USA), the laws are so that you have to seek out information about a natural product separate from the product's packaging. You can do so by asking questions from someone knowledgeable or reading separate literature sources.

Another potential problem is exotic (for you) foods, beverages and herbal medicines, I have an uncle who ate a lot of palm oil while in a foreign country and it stopped up his intestinal system. He developed a very dangerous condition, but the natives regularly use palm oil all their lives.

I use diet and lifestyle for health and healing and try not to use supplements, pharmaceuticals, medicinal herbs or homeopathies. Treatment with strong herbs can lead to bad reactions in a hurry if you are not careful. Any herb or exotic plant must be approached with caution and research before use. A bad reaction can happen in an unexpected way, as everyone's body is different. Some signs of adverse reactions are headache, skin rash, and bloating in the intestinal area. *Any negative effect* on or in the body may be due to an adverse reaction to a supplement, food, herb or medicine. This negative effect may be sudden or grow over a period of time, in days, weeks and longer.

Another personal example, lately I decided to do a harder work out program, lifting weights, rock climbing, and doing more stationary bike workouts. I was pushing myself, so I thought I needed more protein and I decided to try out a vegan protein powder and to eat more fish and egg protein. Things went well with the protein powder drink for about a week.

However, one day I drank a normal dosage of protein powder. My kidneys rebelled, and they started to hurt. I had a lot of thirst that evening and drank about a gallon of water. I had to stop the protein powder, and I took hydrangea herb tincture for a few days to ease the kidneys.

I have decided to back off the intensity of my workouts and eat less protein and pace out my exercise program. I can still get to where I want to, but it will take a little longer. I took the hydrangea herb tincture for about a week. It did help ease my kidneys, but I was getting a headache from the herb, so I went off it.

Another personal example, I used to drink Aloe Vera juice for a health tonic-a little bit every day. However, over a few months I felt that I was not doing very well with this daily drink. I could feel a negative effect, mainly in area of my liver, so I stopped. Nevertheless, I read about people on the internet drinking a little aloe juice daily and my wife's parents take it every day with good effect. However, my digestive system did not like this daily tonic, while others seem to do well. Some of these variations may depend on the quality of the product.

The lesson here is to be careful and listen to your own body as a primary guide. Most people should follow this rule. I think herbals and homeopathies may be useful for short-term treatment, but I am careful of long-term daily tonic usage. Nevertheless, as a counter example my wife uses a mild woman's herbal formula for health on a daily basis with good results. Ultimately, use your own body's response as the final guide in treatments.

It is best to listen to your body while doing exercises, homeopathies, medicines, exotic foods, and herbs, etc. To me this is a correct approach to health, if you push until something breaks, something will, and you may not get health back.

A similar caution with supplements is that they may be fine long term, or harmful, depending on the supplement and how much taken. I personally consider it best in general to use whole food supplements made from foods for any long-term supplementation. Moreover, take the least amount needed. This is an approach for the best chance for long life, and not risk harming organs and prematurely age them.

Personally, I primarily focus on using gentle natural ways in healing. Usually choosing foods and lifestyle over stronger methods, such as strong herbs, supplements and pills, because these often have undesirable side effects. This approach takes more effort and discipline than taking a "magic" pill, supplement or herb.

There is no hard rule in supplementation, herbs, foods, or pills. It is a dance between getting what you need, verses the risk of sickness or damaging the body's organs due to unforeseeable adverse effects.

Chapter Twenty Six

Why buy organic?

From 2006 and onward, honeybees all around the world are disappearing and dying at unprecedented rates. The cause for this is not clear, but may be because of genetically modified plants, herbicides and pesticides in farmer's fields. The bee's diet may be inadequate or harmful in some way. Is it possible domesticated bees are having a hard time living on a modern manmade diet? To me this is another indicator that our food is becoming unhealthier in recent times.

Genetically modified (GM) foods were put on the market in mass starting in the early 1990's. Corn and soy seem to be the GM crops most often used today. These are fed to livestock and are ingredients inside many processed products including corn oil, vegetable oil and corn syrup.

Many countries all across the world have banned or limited GM foods for various reasons. Industry may engineer new traits inside plants, sometimes by adding in genetics from foreign species. For instance, to reduce the need for pesticides they may give the plant an internal pesticide effect. Genetic changes are being made and no doubt, some of these are beneficial in some way. Still, it is a gamble how they will affect long-term health in people.

Food industry creates modified foods and they are tested real time on the population. It is a question, is something harmful and if so, how much? Foods are constantly changing because of genetic modifications, pesticides and food additives. You should keep on top of what is going on. I actually think bees dying off are a good thing in a way, as it should force the food industry to step back. Eating organic and non-processed foods may be even more important in the future for best health. Beware, some foods labeled natural, or organic, may not be truly organic, or natural. They may have pesticides, chemical residues and additives in trace amounts. However, this is more likely with non-organic foods. There are foods labeled organic with canola oil in them. Just because something came out of the health, section of a store does not mean it is healthy; some ordinary store products may be better.

I am not against all genetic modification, but I think the rate of change is too great for safety. Humans for thousands of years ate slowly changing foods in terms of food additives, hormones, herbicides, pesticides, and genetic changes. Today food can be changed from one season to the next. Such rapid changes when and if they occur may cause a bad reaction to a food item you ate fine in the past. It is notable that I can get bad reactions to certain foods that my wife can eat fine, and visa versa.

I have a lot of experience in trying new foods, supplements and herbs. Even when self-monitoring carefully by feeling one's condition, you may still have an eroding health effect that you cannot tell for a long time. Alternatively, one may have a noticeably bad reaction happen quickly.

Food coming in from every corner of the planet is new in human history. A food from another part of the world, your body may have no genetic history with it. Be careful of out of area for you foods and exotic to you foods. Watch out for bad reactions when experimenting with anything new. Be careful of social emersion in a foreign country. A good food for locals may overwhelm your body quickly or may erode health slowly until sickness.

A common food may destroy health because your genetics and lifetime body history are not of the area where you live. Another problem is when growing up we see foreign to our body foods all of our lives. It is hard to tell what may be truly foreign to our bodies in social immersion. For example, in western society, we have an abundance of dairy products, but many people cannot handle dairy. What is common to eat in local culture of today, your body may not recognize as good food.

It is possible to have a slight allergic reaction to a food or supplement, so mild that you can hardly tell it, and what caused it. So pay close attention to how you feel because this will slowly erode health.

As I am writing, I feel hung over this morning but I should feel great. I am thinking I had an adverse reaction to something. I suspect the organic yogurt I ate the night before. I had eaten it again even though I suspected a bad reaction from it the last time. I checked the ingredients and everything looks good, but I do not feel well. Even though it looks fine, I think something is wrong with it for my body. Maybe an unlisted food additive, by the law if an additive is less than one percent; it does not have to be listed in my country. Anyway, I must avoid this product from now on.

If after I eliminated eating this yogurt and I feel bad again, I will reevaluate and try to change something else about my foods or environment. However, from my experience I am certain it is from this specific yogurt product, because similar adverse reactions have happened to me before from other yogurt products. Nevertheless, I do fine with some yogurt products I need more investigation. I wonder if someday all store bought yogurt will give me a bad reaction or only some specific yogurt brands. I wonder if there are ingredients in some yogurt products that are not on the food label. I know I am allergic to non-organic cornstarch, and the bad effect feels like what happens to me when I eat non-organic corn products. I notice some yogurt products have cornstarch on the label used as filler and I avoid these.

Two things that I am aware of, foods are changing all the time, but also my body is changing, as I get older. It is because as people age their digestion system becomes weaker, and toxins build up over time. Therefore, adverse reactions can become stronger and more noticeable. Is it because of a changing food or is my body changing?

Chapter Twenty-Seven
Cooking is a methodology

The aim of this cooking section is to show some general ideas about cooking, rather than a large list of recipes.

For health, there is a general rule, raw foods, sprouted foods and lightly cooked foods are the best choices. Anything processed should be eaten less often. While transitioning toward better health, find the healthier processed foods in the stores such as the healthier cookies, cakes, breads, sodas, candies etc. For best health, it is better to transition away from all processed foods when you are ready. This includes the more healthy versions.

I do eat some processed foods, but I limit them to the healthiest items and I mostly eat foods prepared from scratch. It is better to create palatable home cooked meals from source foods such as beans, grains, vegetables and fruits. I sometimes eat a little store bought yogurt, organic butter, rice based pasta, and healthier versions of cottage cheese. Therefore, I eat some processed foods, but I feel better when I limit them. For the longest healthy lifespan, it is best to eat organic foods raw or cooked from scratch.

Processing of any kind at best destroys nutrition to an extent, or worse, processing may add in preservatives and additives. Additives are to improve taste, shelf life and texture of food, but may cause toxins to build up inside the body. Look at the product labels for food ingredients and you will see a number of unfamiliar chemical names. A lot of processing is hidden, like radiating foods, or using pesticides for shipment. In addition, there are chemical processes to ripen food in the store after being shipped in from overseas. It is best to wash fruit when home, a scrub brush that dispenses soap is effective. Buy organic fruit as much as you can to avoid pesticides. However, even organic fruit may have pesticides on it, but it is usually much less than non-organic.

Foods may have trace amounts of chemicals that are not listed in the ingredients. You have to be careful even of organically labeled processed foods in health food stores. In this changing world, you have to keep on your toes and trust nothing completely. Shipped in organic products is a step up, but local organic produce is often better. Growing it at home is another option. Industry may do harmful processes on food for long distance shipping. Locally grown organic produce in season is least likely to have harmful processes done on it.

The healthy food, fruits and vegetables shipped to your store from long distance out of season have to be picked green then packaged for shipment. Sometimes unhealthy processes are used to give food a pleasing appearance in the store. As you can imagine, it is best to buy local, organic, in season, and grow your own food as much as possible. Frozen raw foods are an option, as they are frozen while fresh and packaged soon after harvesting. I do buy out of area produce trying to find organic as much as I can. Cost is a factor when grocery shopping, do the best you can and grow a garden if you are able.

As a practical manner, I use processed foods such as canned and frozen foods for meals. The best food is fresh organic produce. The second best is frozen foods and third best is canned foods. The worst is any extremely processed food that is quick to eat, or cook then eat.

There are two schools of thought on flavorings. You can eat a diet very plain and simple using few spices and culinary herbs like Biblical Daniel, Shaolin monks and various long-lived mountain peoples. The other way is to spice it up with culinary herbs and spices.

I myself try to make tasty foods without extreme seasoning. Some culinary herbs have a beneficial effect on health. However, I think it best for the organs and body not to over indulge in anything with strong effect, flavor and smell. Any short-term study by science should be weighed against long-term experience of our most healthy ancestors.

For everyday usage, I suggest flavoring foods only to taste, in order to make them palatable. For example, garlic is a healthy culinary herb to cook with, but I would not load lots of garlic into my food every day. If nothing else, you will have a non-social smell on your body. Instead, use garlic to pleasant taste and smell in the appropriate kinds of foods on occasion such as in stir-fries and soups. Hot peppers can be good for people with heart disease, but again I would use it in my food only to taste. You can take garlic and hot pepper supplementation.

Simple tasty cooking does not depend on a cookbook. It depends on a few staple foods and condiments and general knowledge on how to use them. The first step is to obtain this list of supplies.

1. Braggs Aminos: This sauce tastes like soy sauce, and is made up of healthy amino acids.

2. Nutritional yeast: This is a special yeast with a full compliment of B vitamins and is a complete protein. You can find it in health food stores or in the natural food section in many grocery stores. It is very flavorful and an important nutrition source for a vegetarian or low meat eater diet. (Brewers yeast, though very healthy is bitter in taste)

3. Olive oil and safflower oil: I suggest getting olive oil made in Europe, because they have strict laws about producing healthy cold pressed oil. Select cold pressed when available for any kind of oil, avoid expeller pressing as it causes damaging heat in the oil. Olive oil is good for salads and low temperature cooking; safflower oil is good for higher temperature cooking. Neither is genetically modified as far as I know. However, safflower oil has a short fifty-year history in human usage. Other good oils to consider are grape seed, walnut, avocado, sunflower and sesame seed.

I use olive oil as my primary oil, because it has several thousand years of use in human history. Olive oil has a very good long-term history backing up its usage. It seems that industry is working toward genetically modifying everything these days and this practice is increasing, I am suspicious of most oils so I am very careful in restaurants. Hydrogenated oil is particularly bad, and its usage these days seems to be declining. However, industry may be replacing the hydrogenated oil with other additives or processes that are as harmful. Canola oil is being used more often and vegetable oil with soy, corn, and cotton seed oil in it. All of these are genetically modified. Ingesting suspect oils may be harmful to health over time.

4. Raw nuts and seeds: Buy walnuts, pecans, almonds, cashews, pumpkin seeds, sunflower seeds, chia seeds and sesame seeds. Roasted nuts are not healthy because the heat during roasting changes the molecular structure of the nut's oil. Raw nuts are good food, but be careful of over eating them and gaining an allergy. A sign of allergy reaction are spots of itchy skin anywhere on the body. A tiny handful of each a day is about right. Nuts are not conducive to dieting due to fat content. Some salt in nuts is fine, but avoid roasted salted nuts and limit nuts and seeds with fancy flavorings for long-term health. I consider nuts and seeds to be a very important source for protein, healthy fat and nutrition.

5. Sea salt: It has minerals in it. Buying sea salt with iodine is good.

6. Organic butter: I use it to lightly flavor foods and on toasted bread at times. Avoid excessive usage for health.

7. Organic chicken stock: I consider the vegetarian kind the best.

8. Culinary Herbs: These are for flavoring and health, and are used only to taste; black pepper (use black pepper sparingly), garlic powder, onion powder, and cayenne powder.

9. Onions, garlic and hot peppers: Buy fresh as needed and use to taste.

10. Veganaise: Buy or make this type of healthy mayonnaise, it is better for health than common mayonnaise. (Recipe at end of chapter)

11. Pimento cheese: You make this healthy cheese spread yourself. (Recipe at end of chapter)

12. Non-GMO lecithin: This is a type of fat,

most often made from soybeans. Buy lecithin made from non-GMO sources. Lecithin helps the brain and nervous system function well, and helps keep veins and arteries clean. Lecithin is an emulsification fat that puts other fats into suspension.

I use lecithin, garlic, and cayenne pepper as natural treatment to help keep my heart and arteries clean. I use lecithin all the time for my heart. I take a spoonful or two during the day, most days. At times, I may take more lecithin to help clean up my arteries due to eating things that I should not have.

Staple foods are potatoes, beans and rice, such as brown, jasmine or wild rice. My wife likes the short grain brown rice or jasmine rice, as they are quicker to cook. Eat any kind of fruit or vegetable, fresh or frozen, another staple food is oats. Frozen foods are particularly good, as the freezing happens when they are fresh. The freezing process does some damage, but it is acceptable.   Canned food is fine, avoiding additives and sugar, but fresh and frozen foods are better.

Common staple foods that should be limited are pastas and breads. Any common type of processed modern store bought bread might have too much yeast and additives that are not healthy. Bread made in Biblical times was dense and made with course grain, with no preservatives or additives and little yeast in it. Modern commercially made bread is not the same as bread made in Biblical days. I do eat modern bread, spaghetti sauce and rice pasta, but in limited amounts. My wife is allergic to dairy products and I often do not feel good when eating dairy or store bought breads. We limit eating dairy to a little yogurt, cottage cheese and butter.

Gluten is the sticky part of grains. My wife is allergic to gluten so we avoid it. When I eat a lot of pasta, pizza or bread containing wheat, my belly and intestines do not feel well. I think many people have an adverse reaction to high gluten content processed foods and do not realize it. I buy pasta that is rice based or another kind of low gluten containing pasta. Some people decide to go on a health diet and restrict meat and then eat much gluten filled meat replacement products. I think this practice is unhealthy. I believe clean meat is healthier than gluten filled meat replacement products.

My wife as a young girl did not have chewing gum, so as kids will do, she and friends invented chewing gum. Her mother had bags of wheat and they found if they chewed it long enough that it would turn into balls of gluten. Gluten chews like gum and can even blow bubbles! They even used balls of this gluten gum to temporarily repair holes in their old rowboat!

When people eat processed pastas, breads and cakes and then feel sick most will blame gluten because it is the popular item of today to blame. They assume gluten is the cause. However, there are other possibilities. Many additives are in common breads and cakes. There is a lectin allergy, which overlaps foods that contain gluten. In addition, excessive yeast can be inside bread, because many types of bread have high yeast content during processing. High yeast content in finished bread products can make you sick. This can happen in homemade breads as well.

Even the more healthy commercially made breads can be harmful. If you like bread, then find naturally made breads with no additives and low in yeast content such as sourdough or salt rising bread. Natural bread will spoil more quickly if left out, because of no additives. Health may dramatically improve when eating better quality bread and cutting out bad breads and cakes, or eating no bread at all. The benefit may be slow to happen, so be patient when experimenting. It may take six weeks to get gluten out of achy joints and feel a large benefit.

Canned foods without any added preservatives or additives are fine. Although, I consider it best to buy fresh foods, then frozen, and then lastly canned products. Caution, regular can openers put bits of metal into the food. Better is the can openers that cut the top edge of the can, and then can use the top as a lid. To understand the need, use a magnet after you open a can with a regular can opener; sweep out the bits of metal and look at them!

Regarding corn, these days I can only eat organic corn because in the last decade some non-organic corn products make me sick. I suspect the cause is due to genetically engineered toxins inside some kinds of corn in order to control insects. Even if you have no noticeable bad effect from corn, it may be a good idea to buy organic corn products.

Breakfast

A favorite breakfast for health is oatmeal. Procedure, find two small glasses the same size, one is for water, the other for oats, fill one two times with water and put the water in the cooking pot. Then fill the other once with oats, do not put the oats in the pot yet. This creates two parts water, one part oats. Then in the water shake in a little sea salt and add in a little oil, maybe half a teaspoon. Bring the water to boil then add in oats, turn down heat to the lowest setting and cook until done. This simple procedure will work for rice and most any other grain.

After the oats are done I add fruit, nuts and raw seeds, (I may add a little milk product, this makes it more tasty, but may be less healthy), lecithin on top is very healthy. You can use any cooked grain for breakfast. Some choices are quinoa, millet, buckwheat, rice and hominy. Consider mixing bran into the grain for more nutrition. I do not use premade breakfast foods, it is better to make breakfast from scratch. Do not microwave water to boiling and dump it into the grain; the food will not cook completely even with quick oats.

I currently like rice or oatmeal the best for breakfast. They are common, healthy, inexpensive, and cook up in a few minutes. We have tried various different milks, oatmeal milk, coconut milk, soymilk and almond milk. Almond milk seems the best for us. All milk is processed, so no milk at all can be the healthiest option. However, this is up to the individual because some milk is nice in cereal.

My wife occasionally makes pancakes or waffles for breakfast from organic non-gluten flour. She mixes in blueberries or other fruit and uses pure maple syrup on top along with frozen fruit. I personally find there are several flours that cause me to have adverse reactions. Some of these are the so-called healthy flours from the health food store. I have to test all flours by trial and error. I actually feel fine with ordinary white flour. These days I avoid most flours and breads because I feel better without them.

The healthier option for bread is the Biblical kinds of breads. Soughdough bread with the least processed flours is another option. Local bakery breads should have no additives, be sure to ask about the flour. Local baked bread is harder to find, but it is often worth the effort for health.

Sometimes, we have salad for breakfast, spinach greens along with other vegetables, then olive oil and lemon juice as condiments. Add a small dollop of cottage cheese and put on raw seeds. Alternatively, you may have a breakfast salad with real body. It is made with layers of greens and other vegetables, avocados, tomatoes, with cooked beans and brown rice inside or on the side. This is a haystack. It is great fun to make a haystack for kids because they love the name.

On occasion, we will have an evening type meal for breakfast made of leftovers. At times, I like an egg sandwich made with healthy bread. I like to have runny eggs and add on onions and tomatoes. I spread veganaise on the bread for taste and nutrition.

Do not be restricted to traditional breakfast foods, you can juice, have leftovers, or eat most anything that is healthy. Some traditional American breakfast foods are not that healthy. Bacon, sausage and greasy foods may be eaten on rare occasions, while choosing the healthiest versions possible. Replace the pork source of bacon and sausage with healthier alternatives such as turkey. Eggs are healthy, but for most people it is best not to exceed around four to five eggs week. Excessive egg eating may create an allergic or addictive food reaction to eggs and may raise cholesterol and blood pressure.

When boiling soup and other vegetables add sea salt and oil to the water with the vegetables while cooking, the amount varies. Normally I just shake the saltshaker for a little bit and put in about a teaspoon to a tablespoon of oil. Use taste and dietary needs to gauge amount. A very large pot of soup needs more sea salt to get the taste right. Any healthy oil is acceptable to use, including flax oil, walnut oil, grape seed oil, and olive oil. It is best to add salt, and oil while cooking, not after, I find that flavor and digestion is better.

Lunch

If you are following two meals a day diet program, then lunch is easy. Just some fruit, vegetables, nuts, seeds, and a glass of fruit juice or anything else healthy and light. This snack lunch is variable. It can be very small with a single piece of fruit or more as you need.

Remember, lunch is only raw foods on a two meals a day program.

How to eat raw foods between the two main meals depends on your needs. You can snack several times midday with raw foods. Alternatively, eat a raw foods meal at lunchtime or even eat no midday snack at all, it is up to you.

The stricter you are with eating two meals, the better it works for dieting. For best health, do-not over eat, and let your organs rest in between meals. This rest can be two times a day or one time a day, depending on your eating habits. Honestly, I snack lightly midday. I eat raw foods and let my digestion organs rest overnight. I have no trouble maintaining current body weight, as I am active with decent metabolism. Although to lose weight I would have to cut out midday snacking, or increase exercise. Alternatively, I can change the types of foods eaten midday by choosing *only* low fat and low glycemic index foods, such as raw fruits and vegetables even avoiding nuts, seeds and dried fruits.

For a meal type of lunch, you can pack an avocado sandwich. It is a sliced up avocado with tomato and onion with veganaise smoothed out on the insides of the bread. Alternatively, make a raw almond butter and preserves sandwich, or make an onion tomato sandwich with veganaise. If you want to avoid bread then pack some containers of cooked food from home.

Always carry organic apples and other fresh fruits such as bananas and oranges. A tasty snack is a bag of small sweet peppers that can be found in grocery stores. Sweet peppers are high in vitamin C. In order to feel satisfied at a meal, you need to think of proteins, fats and carbohydrates in a combination. Try to pack healthy forms of each of these from low processed sources. This means avoiding cakes, pastries and candy bars.

For example, I normally carry in my car a can of green olives in sea salt. This gives me healthy fat and carbohydrate, and I sometimes like drinking some of the salt water out of the can. Look for canned olives packed in sea salt for best health or those packed in healthy vinegar.

I may have a boiled egg, with a container of leftover beans and rice with a dollop of Veganaise in top. Veganaise is full of healthy fat. I do not buy Veganaise made with canola oil.

Dinner

The daily goal is a healthy home cooked meal with excess food for leftovers, then cycle the leftovers back through for quick meals later on.

Healthy quick evening meals are easy. At the start of the week, cook a big pot of beans and store in the refrigerator. Alternatively, you may use organic canned beans for convenience. Just open a can when needed, any kind of bean is good food. Cook up a big pot of brown rice. This is a staple food to last all week, beans and rice is a complete protein source. In addition, you may cook up a large pot of potatoes for the week as another staple food. Other options are large pots of soup or stew loaded with healthy vegetables and a little meat-if any. The idea here is to store up cooked staple foods in the refrigerator for the rest of the week. In addition, when you cook any extra food will be ingredients for quick meals later on.

As you can tell, the staples are potatoes, beans and rice, to cook these for a week's supply at the start of the week. We buy many frozen vegetables and use them when needed. For condiments we mainly use oil, nutritional yeast, salt and Braggs Amino, add these in while cooking. At serving time put a dollop of Veganaise on top of the beans and rice. You can steam cook vegetables, or stir-fry them in a bit of oil.

This is an example of a good simple meal, beans, brown rice, potatoes and vegetables with a healthy salad on the side. Most food needs salting while cooking, not afterward. It is better to cook salt inside the food because it has much better flavor when you salt to taste while cooking. A bit of salt used when cooking is better for flavor than a large amount of salt on top afterward. Most food needs oil to taste better. Add it in while cooking for best flavor and health.

The best salad in the world is very simple. Use herb greens and spinach (spinach is sweet), then add in sliced sweet peppers, carrots, tomatoes, and any other vegetables as you desire. The dressing is healthy oil and lemon juice or apple cider vinegar. Throughout the salad are raw pumpkin and sunflower seeds. An important item for health and taste is one or two ripe sliced avocados in the salad. For more protein, add in cooked beans. This salad can be a whole meal or a side item.

Lecithin goes well on any canned sliced fruit dish or in any cooked grain breakfast, for example on peaches and oatmeal. Nutritional yeast goes well in most cooked vegetables and grains, for example with pasta, beans, potatoes and rice. Nutritional yeast with butter and sea salt tastes great in popcorn. (I eat popcorn only as an occasional treat because I often feel sluggish the day after eating it.)

Simple vegetable soup, or as I call it "Man Soup" is good for health. Use fresh or frozen vegetables of all kinds, such as broccoli, kale, brussel sprouts, onions, carrots, cabbage and sea weed, anything that looks good in a soup. Chop it all up into a giant pot. Add salt, you may add healthy vegetable base stock, put in Braggs Amino Acids and nutritional yeast, and pore in a little oil. Then taste it, making sure you have enough salt, but not too much. I like to throw in a few handfuls of cooked rice to give it more body, this is optional, no meat in my soup. Cook for about thirty minutes, then enjoy. Save the leftovers for later. Drink the soup broth for best health-if it is not too salty.

For quick meals later on in the week, you have leftovers, rice, potatoes and beans stored in the refrigerator. In addition, you can make a salad and cook some steamed or boiled vegetables. You can make a healthy meal in about fifteen minutes or less using leftovers. Practice using the condiments on the list I gave and your meals will be tasty, healthy and quick.

A large skillet with a lid works well for leftovers. Put in a bit of healthy oil or water and cook the food at a moderate temperature until it is warm. Leftovers are very tasty when warmed in this way. You may sauté' (fry gently) as you like, depending on the type of leftover. Substitute oil with a bit of water if you are dieting. Water works best in a non-stick pan. Do not make it a habit of warming up foods in a microwave; it is a danger for health. The microwave changes the molecular structure of the food. Do not use old aluminum pots for cooking. Excessive aluminum in the body will cause health problems, only use the best modern cookware. It is healthier to use silver or silver-coated silverware. All of my silverware is silver or silver coated. Most of it bought cheaply from second hand stores.

We have an electric pressure cooker that cooks up anything in quick order. Start the timer, and then do not worry about it. In addition, we have a small convection oven with a timer, and an electric wok. Doing other tasks while cooking with these is worry free. I suggest at the least to obtain a wok and use it for healthy meals.

A favorite is egg sandwiches for breakfast or other meals. They are quick and easy, just an egg, veganaise and whatever else you like in a sandwich. If avoiding bread, eat eggs with rice.

If you notice the food selection, the core staples are simple natural foods. The secret, if there is one, is how to use a few tasty healthy condiments with simple foods. Buy the list of condiments that I recommend and learn how to use them and you will have tasty simple meals that cook up quickly.

Snacks

It is harder to have quick snacks when cooking most things from scratch. However, if you concentrate on raw foods for snacks it gets easier. We have fruit, such as an organic apple, but likely you are still hungry after such a snack. It is because there is no protein or fat in fruit or raw vegetables. Therefore, add some raw nut butters or raw nuts, or grab a can of olives packed in sea salt or an avocado in order to obtain fat and protein. Avoid processed snacks, even the healthier items from a health food store if you want to be as healthy as possible and lose weight. Of course when transitioning toward better health habits, it is fine to eat processed snacks when needed.

The snacks I like are a big spoonful of lecithin, apples, bananas, and homemade fruit juice popsicles. If I am hungry, I may have a leftover homemade organic cornbread muffin with preserves and raw almond butter. As you can tell if I am home, I do rummage around for leftovers. I do this when my second meal is running late and I am hungry. In the car, I usually carry a lunch box filled with raw fruit, canned green olives and raw nuts/seeds and dried fruit. It is better to go for these rather than just buying anything at a convenience store-when starving and running late in the day.

For health, try not to snack after the last evening meal, prevent all late night snacking. However, if you do, go for fruit or a glass of fruit juice, anything easy to digest. On this program, most people will be a little hungry before going to bed. This is good, as it implies the digestion organs will rest overnight. The body can concentrate more on healing, not bloated and digesting. The evening meal should be no later than around 6 pm on average. When you wake up in the morning you should feel hungry and not bloated, if full you ate too much the day before.

To be able to get through the long time in between the morning meal and evening meal it is important to fill up on low glycemic index foods for breakfast. Use foods that digest and release energy slowly. They last longer than high glycemic index foods.

If you find yourself off your health program today, get back on it tomorrow. It is not the end of the world. It is all right to have an occasional healthy treat in the late evening. I find it best for myself not to bring harmful treats home, to leave them in the store. If you have bad foods at home, do not feel you must eat them, throw them away.

It is best to eat natural source foods as much as possible. Just one bad processed item on a regular basis may destroy health. For example, lately I notice I have been eating too much cheese. On rare occasions a bit of cheese is fine for me. However, when I eat too much, it clogs my arteries. When so, I eat extra lecithin and get away from cheese.

Recipes

Pimento Cheese Sauce

½ cup distilled water
¼ tsp. garlic powder
¾ cup Raw cashew pieces
½ cup pimentos (do not drain)
3 Tbsp. Nutritional Yeast flakes
1 Tbsp. lemon Juice
¼ tsp. sea salt
1 tsp. dill weed
2 tsp. onion powder

In a blender, combine the water and nuts. Blend until smooth then add in rest of ingredients and blend until creamy. Use as a cheese spread on bread, on cooked rice noodles or you may bake into foods such as potatoes.

Veganaise
1 cup safflower oil
1 ½ tsp salt
1 box of "Mori-Nu Tofu Firm"
½ tsp garlic powder
1 Tbsp apple cider vinegar
½ tsp onion powder
2 Tbsp brown rice syrup
3 Tbsp lemon juice

Blend until creamy, much cheaper than store bought veganaise. Use as a spread on bread and put dollops of it on beans and rice. You can use it like regular mayonnaise.

Best Oat Burgers
Pre heat oven to 375 degrees F, serves twelve.

4 ½ cups water
½ cup Braggs Aminos
¼ cup olive oil
1 Tbsp onion powder
1 ½ tsp garlic powder
1 Tbsp ground sage
4 tsp honey
½ cup yeast flakes

Combine the above ingredients together and bring to a boil. Add 4 ½ cups of quick oats (may substitute a part of quick oats with oat bran for more nutrition) then boil for two minutes. Scoop onto cookie sheet and inside wide mouth Mason jar rings. Remove rings and bake for thirty minutes on each side (one hour total time baking). These veggie burgers are better than any I have found from the super market. Put excess in freezer. They also taste great with gravy on top, or break them up to make meatballs for rice spaghetti.

Chapter Twenty-Eight
More on oil and fat

Selecting healthy oil can be a difficult problem because there is so much conflicting information. As a start, cold pressed olive oil is healthy. Cold pressing has no damaging heat. I would stay away from canola oil. Its history is short and it is a genetic creation from the rape seed plant. I would avoid vegetable oils because they can be made from canola, cottonseed, soy and corn, all of these may be genetically modified. We do use safflower oil because it is affordable oil and can cook with it at higher temperature. I use quality olive oil as first choice and any other oil in a lesser amount. Other very good oils are almond, sesame, avocado, walnut, grape seed and sunflower.

Coconut oil and palm oil may be used for high temperature cooking, but personally, I am cautious about using them. They are solid at room temperature, so it follows they may be harder to digest. They may be fine for you, especially if your family has a positive genetic history with their use. It also depends on how much you ingest.

A true story, a friend with Scandinavian ancestry went overseas to Borneo many years ago. The natives used abundant local palm oil for everything, but for him it eventually clogged up his digestive system, a dangerous condition. A doctor removed part of his intestine to clean it out. The natives use this oil extensively all their lives.

Watch out for olive oil combined with other oil in restaurants such as canola oil and still called olive oil. When you eat out in restaurants bad oil can cause ill health over time. One can select otherwise healthy items, but bad cooking oil may harm health. There is no long-term human history with many modern day oils. In restaurants, I avoid oily or deep fried foods. Generally, home cooking with fresh organic produce and good oil is the safest practice. Restaurants are not going to use expensive healthy oils because it costs too much. They tend to use oils from genetically engineered plants, and oils made by less healthy processes. Restaurants will hide the use of cheaper oils. Remember oil is inside most everything, including pastries.

My personal experience is that canola has become popular in the last few years in my local restaurants and in processed foods. The most popular oil in your home area restaurants may be different. The popular oils used in processed foods can vary in time, so keep checking food labels. Why would the oils used in food change? People may force change if enough get sick and therefore refuse to buy bad products. Industry may change oil if forced to by government because too many people are getting sick. Alternatively, newer, even cheaper oils may come on the market.

I eat out during social events. This is fine on occasion. Otherwise, it is best to eat at home with family. Eating out may support a happier lifestyle for a single person. Balance out lifestyle choices the best you can, healthy social interaction verses healthy eating. In restaurants, choose steam cooking and baking when given a choice. You may bring along a small container of healthy oil and condiments.

For home use, buy cold pressed oils. A good choice is olive oil from Europe. The second choice would be expeller pressed oil. Expeller pressing creates heat, which changes the molecular structure of the oil. Avoid oils that are chemically extracted, because industry often cannot remove all chemicals used for extraction. To avoid chemically extracted oil, use oils that say *cold pressed, this* is best, or *expeller pressed*. Otherwise, assume the oil is chemically extracted. If CO_2 gas is used as the extraction chemical, it can be removed, but often manufacturers use the chemical hexane, which can leave traces.

Of course, avoid hydrogenated oil and avoid most butter substitutes because they usually have unhealthy oils in concentration. I prefer using organic butter to any butter substitute that I have seen. No other cooking oil has a longer positive human history than cold pressed olive oil, so I use it as my primary oil.

For home cooking, you should not deep-fry anything. It is better to sauté, to sauté, put a little oil in a skillet and then lightly cook food. You can warm up leftovers in a covered skillet using olive oil or water while using moderate temperature. You should not let the heat build to the smoking point this makes the oil toxic. Avoid or limit deep fried foods at home and when eating out.

In ancient times, most people ate a better ratio of Omega 3 fats verses Omega 6 fats. Today many people do not get enough Omega 3 rich oils. High amounts of Omega 3 is found in fish oil, flax seed oil, soy oil, walnut oil and walnuts. Farm animals raised on grass have a higher amount of Omega 3 fatty acids than farm animals fattened with grains. The same for fish, fish farm fish have less Omega 3 fats than wild ocean fish, unless Omega 3 fats are included in their food. To obtain more Omega 3 fatty acids you can eat fish or walnuts or quality walnut oil. Omega 3 rich eggs are in some stores. Free-range chickens have up to two times more Omega 3 fat than cage-raised chickens.

Omega 3 fatty acids are very beneficial for health. Olive oil has a ten to one ratio of Omega 6 fatty acid to Omega 3 fatty acid, which is considered adequate. Recent research suggests that a five to one ratio is better. I suggest eating some high Omega 3 fatty acid foods. Both Omega 3 and Omega 6 fatty acids are essential, which means the body cannot make them, so you must consume each on a regular basis.

To calculate daily oil consumption, we can use the average caloric intake for men and women. The average daily calories for men should be about 2500 a day, for women about 2000 a day. If you want 25% to 35% of calories in fat, how can you estimate this in a practical way? Without counting fat in everything, and if you mostly eat home cooked foods and some raw nuts and seeds. First off, we assume that we are getting about half of daily fat requirements from nuts, seeds and other natural resources such as avocados. Therefore, we need to figure out how much olive oil to add in food for each person to make up the rest.

There are 13.5 grams of fat and 120 calories per tablespoon of olive oil. Twenty-five percent of 2500 calories is 625 calories, 35% of 2500 calories is 875 calories. Taking half of these numbers will give 312 and 437 calories respectively. This means 2.6 to 3.6 tablespoons of olive oil a day to be added into food for the average man. For the average woman it adds up to 2 to 2.9 tablespoons of olive oil a day. These numbers assume that you are eating 1/2 of daily fat in nuts, seeds, olives and avocados, etc.

A whole cup of mixed raw nuts and seeds can supply half to a hundred percent of daily needed fat (54 grams) on average. If you want to lose weight, watch how many nuts, butter and fat you eat. If you are ingesting plenty of fat from other sources, cut down oil used in cooking. Fat in the diet is easily converted to fat on the body. If you are having trouble losing weight, reduce fat in your diet and increase intake of low glycemic pulse foods.

Note: a tablespoon of butter has about 70 calories, which is about half of olive oil. A single olive has about four fat calories. A regular sized can of olives will have about 220 fat calories. A full size avocado has about 20 to 30 grams of fat, which is about 195 fat calories.

For homework look up oils, individual nuts, seeds, other fat sources, and crunch the numbers for your own diet.

Chapter Twenty-Nine
Human history of common foods

If we are serious about being healthy, we need to think about the long-term history of food. Are our bodies designed to eat all foods from everywhere on earth? The evidence says no. In a region, people are adapted to a selection of foods that people living in a different area may not be able to tolerate. People should think about where they genetically come from before eating any kind of food.

Examples are coconuts and palms, what people have a long-term history of ingesting these? Europeans do not have a long history with these, as compared to the tropical island dwellers. This makes it more likely they will have an adverse reaction. How about milk products, what is the long-term human history with this food. What regions had dairy foods several hundred years ago? For instance, the Americas did not have dairy products before the Europeans came.

What about the new foods that are genetically created by humankind? Do we have a long-term human history with these? What are your thoughts about the chemically made preservatives and additives to improve texture, taste, and shelf life? What is our long-term human history with these?

Let us consider safety considerations by regulation agencies in relation to the average human lifespan. Let us say the average person lives to seventy some years of age. From this, regulators can gauge the build up of toxic residues and reactions to them by the average person. However, in a group of people, there can be varied responses to any substance. Some can handle it fine while others may have adverse reactions from trace amounts. The likelihood of adverse reactions happening greatly increases when people are ingesting foods they have little family history of eating.

For example, what is the history of milk usage in your family? Did they have cows in the Americas many hundreds years ago? Did they have cows in the world's tropical islands? The answer is no. Today about 75% of Native Americans are lactose intolerant and about 90% of Asian Americans are lactose intolerant. People with European ancestry have a longer human history with milk, so are less likely to have bad reactions as adults. Most people are able to ingest milk at a younger age and later on lose the ability. People of European decent are more likely to be able to digest milk as adults because of their family history with dairy. The same kind of situation can be with any food, beverage or environmental item.

Many foods fall into a category of a short-term human history, for some or all people and can cause adverse reactions. Some common symptoms are intestinal gas, bloating, stomach pain, nausea, headache, joint pain, and rashes. Any kind of pain or discomfort may be caused by a food intolerance or allergic reaction. It can be a combination of symptoms or just one alone.

Here is a list of common food allergens, or intolerance foods: egg, fish and shellfish, dairy allergies and lactose intolerance, peanuts or any other nuts, sesame seeds, soy, wheat and gluten. It is my experience that you can have strong allergies that you can notice easily. In addition, you may have others that are hard to tell, but are eroding health.

People from Europe have a longer human history with milk products. In contrast, people from tropical areas have a longer human history with native fauna, such as palms and coconuts. If your personal family history is not of a local area where a food item is grown, the likelihood of a bad reaction is higher. Different countries have their own geographic human food history, so each will have their own specific list of most common allergen foods. Here is a list of a few allergen foods.

1.   Corn, originating in the Americas, sent back to Europe around 1500. It has a short human history for non Native American people. It is a genetically engineered crop. I myself only can safely eat organic corn products. I may become ill for several days from eating a lot of a regular processed corn product such as cornbread. Corn has many kinds of uses including corn oil and corn syrup. There is no long-term human history with GMO processed corn products.

2.   Cow's milk was developed for human usage in North West Europe. It has a shorter human history most everywhere else. Bad

reactions from dairy products are common, especially for older adults. Many people can safely eat one or more of these, cottage cheese, yogurt and organic butter. However, be aware that a slight adverse reaction may be happening, that you can hardly tell and is eroding health.

3.   Chocolate has a long history of usage in Central and South America. It was introduced to Europe in the 1500's. It has a short human history for non Native Americans.

4.   Coffee originated in Africa, and it did not gain much acceptance in the Middle East and Europe as a drink until after the 1600's, therefore it has a somewhat short human history of usage. Caffeine has no food value, but it is addictive and may be used as a medicine short term. It may be helpful for migraines, constipation and for staying awake-to a limited degree.

5.   Wheat originated in the Middle East. It is the first crop that allowed civilization because it can be grown and stored in large quantity. It is a great food source, but be careful of concentrated gluten in processed wheat products. People not of that region and surrounding area are more likely to have an allergic reaction to wheat or gluten. An adverse reaction is very possible for most grain products, a notable exception is rice. If you have digestion problems with beans and grains it may be helpful to soak them before cooking, also consider fermenting and sprouting.

6.   Soy originated in Asia and historically used little as a food staple. In recent years, soy usage

has greatly increased worldwide. Currently the primary way to extract soy protein and soy oil is chemically using hexane. Trace amounts of hexane are present in foods after processing. Industry is currently switching to less toxic processing chemicals. Given its short human history as a staple item and genetic engineering, I would be cautious of heavy soy usage. It is best to buy organic soy products.   I eat tofu in moderate amounts and consider it good food.

7.   Potatoes have an ancient history in South America and they were introduced to North America and Europe around 1600. Potatoes are rarely cause adverse reactions, except for people with rheumatoid arthritis. Anyone with arthritis may need to avoid the nightshade family of plants including potatoes. Anyone without genetic history from South American is more likely to have a bad reaction. People concerned about health should eat more red or sweet potatoes than white potatoes. Potatoes are middle to high range in the glycemic index, so you may want to be moderate their use if you are overweight or diabetic. Sweet potatoes are also middle range to high in glycemic index. There are many variables regarding the glycemic index of potatoes, depending on the kind of potato and preparation. For instance, the glycemic index of boiled potatoes is around half of baked. Study the subject how to cook potatoes for the lowest glycemic index if you are diabetic or overweight.

From this short list, we can see that foreign foods are shipped all around the world. In addition, people move all around the world and new foods and beverages are endlessly being created with additives and genetic engineering. When considering foods, it is best to think about their history in relation to personal family history, to prevent adverse reactions. One will hear from friends and experts about new wonderful exotic foods and concentrated extracts, which are healthy. Nevertheless, be cautious and let how you feel be the guide when experimenting.

Thinking of myself, I have a family ancestry of native North American and European decent. I consider myself lucky because my family food history is broad, which enables me to handle a spectrum of natural foods.

The best Biblical Daniel diet is compatible with your own genetic history with meals made from organic pulse foods, with water being the primary beverage.

Chapter Thirty

Parasites and worms

The first step in a health program can be a parasite and worm removal cleanse. Most farmers and pet owners regularly worm their animals. At the same time, most people think it strange that anyone would suggest such a thing for themselves and their children. Really, does this attitude make sense when you think about it? Children are around animals, dirt, and all kinds of unclean items. It is possible that they have parasites and if not eliminated, these will survive into their adult lives. Even adults may become infected with worms and parasites from undercooked meat and other contamination.

It is less likely that adults in modern western society will have parasite infections, but it is possible. It is a mistake to think all parasite infections have strong acute symptoms. A parasite infection may affect health negatively over many years. Parasites may harm joints, organs and digestion. Younger people with a strong immune system may be able to shrug off these negative effects for years. Nevertheless, over time as they get older and their immune system gets weaker, they can become sicker and sicker due to parasites.

How many people have a parasite cleanse and how many people have chronic health problems-especially in the older years? How many health problems are due to parasites in modern society?

A common health problem arises when people take in toxins by foods or from the environment. First, the human body tries to eliminate all toxins by removing them out of the system. If the body cannot do this because of the type of toxin or too much toxin overwhelming the system, then it will store toxins somewhere, often in the body fat in and around organs. (It could be around the reproductive organs for women). If this happens, the immune system can be weaker in that area of the body, if so parasites may migrate there and live.

Cysts may form in a toxin-laden area of the body. A cyst can be a sack or shell with a parasite inside it, and then cancer may start in this area. This process toward illness can take many years, even decades. The first step could have been a child ingesting a parasite many years ago when playing in a yard or stream, or eating undercooked meat, or by being around infected pets, animals or other infected children. Be sure to worm pets on a regular basis and wash hands every time when petting an animal or dealing with pet bedding, vomit or feces. Here is a short list of some common parasites.

1.   Blastocystosis infects about 2% to 20% of the population. Exposure to feces from another infected human or animal spreads infection. There are many kinds of parasite species with corresponding effects or no effect at all depending on the person's genetics and the species. Possible symptoms include general

digestive illness, depression, weakness and joint pain.

2.   Dientamoebiasis infects up to about 10% of the population of industrialized countries. The feces of an infected animal or a human spread the infection. There are different species that may or may not give acute symptoms of illness. Acute symptoms include weakness, nausea, vomiting, and fever.

3.   Toxoplasmosis Parasitic Pneumonia infects up to 33% of all humans worldwide, about 11% in the USA. Infections are from undercooked meat (pork), raw milk, from soil, water or feces of infected animals. A primary host is cats. When first infected flu like symptoms happen, then fade away. Then no symptoms until later on-when the immune system gets weaker for any reason. It commonly attacks the brain and eyes, but it can affect any part of the body.

4.   Human Whipworm is a somewhat rare infection in the USA, but it is thought about 2.2 million are infected in the southeast. About one billion people are infected worldwide. A hundred worms or less inside the body will cause no symptoms. A higher number of worms may cause diarrhea, blood loss and even rectal collapse.

There are many more kinds of parasitic infections than this short list. We see from the statistics parasites are common even in modern society.

Thankfully, it is easy to deal with this potential health problem. Go to any health food store and ask about a full spectrum parasite cleanse formula. I personally like to take an herbal capsule formula of wormwood, cloves and black walnut hull. These three herbs together kill parasites at all stages of life. I buy a full bottle and take as directed until the capsules are gone.

Alternatively, you can get these three herbs in tincture form and take as directed on the bottle. Or you can take a single large dose of one teaspoon of this tincture combination on an empty stomach to remove parasites, but be careful because it will make you feel sick. Consult with a health care provider.

If you have any kind of chronic illness, it is a good first step to consider a parasite cleanse. Then do a parasite removal program ever so often, possibly every year or two as a maintenance program. Consider doing a parasite cleanse program for every family member, even if everyone seems healthy. Taking strong herbal treatments for parasites on a daily basis is not recommended. Here is a list of foods that may be used continuously against parasites.

1.   Aloe Vera juice can be taken on a regular basis by some people. It is antiparasitic. Other people cannot depending on the person and quality of juice. I personally would cycle on and off in its usage.

2.   Raw Garlic kills parasites effectively. Raw garlic is very strong, so be careful. I once juiced a

few cloves and drank it. This is very hard on the stomach and I stopped the practice.

3.   Strong spices such as hot peppers, turmeric, cloves, nutmeg, horseradish, cardamom, cinnamon are effective against parasites. I would be cautious about excessive long-term usage of strong spices. Be careful while experimenting because they can make you sick if eaten in excess.

4.   Coconut Oil has lauric acid that when digested inside the body creates a substance that kills parasites, yeasts and viruses in the gut. Before extensive usage of coconut oil, consider your family history to determine if your body can effectively process it. Monitor how you feel while ingesting.

5.   Pineapple contains the enzyme bromelain, which is antiparasitic.

Of this list, I eat hot peppers, cooked garlic and raw pineapple, all on a semiregular basis. In addition, hot peppers may help with heart and circulatory diseases. By helping to clean the gunk out of arteries and increasing circulation.

Chapter Thirty One

Elimination diet program

Do you have any chronic illness or nagging problem that will not go away? A symptom that gets worse then better, back and forth with no cause and effect that you can tell. If so, there is a good chance it is because of food allergies or food intolerances. There are two ways to deal with this in an elimination diet program. One way is to remove the most suspected food or environmental chemical items one at a time and see how the body reacts. The other way is to remove all suspected items at the same time.

A common problem with an elimination-testing program is that many people cannot pay attention to their body's reactions, and feel cause and effect. I often have to help family members with this, as they are unable to feel their body and remember cause and effect.

A difficult problem is dealing with children with allergies. If a child is chronically sick, one should check and eliminate any possible adverse reaction source. For instance, for a child with a breathing problem, I would start in their bedroom and the whole household, looking for any possible source of chemical or biological toxin that is causing illness. I would check for mold, or chemical fumes off manmade items such as foam products. I would check all chemical products, such as soaps, medicines and household cleaners.

I would make sure their bedding is hypoallergenic, removing dust mites and putting on antidust mite sheets and pillowcases. I would buy an air filter system to put in the house and their bedroom. If you cannot resolve the allergen source, consider taking the child to another location for a time, maybe even to another part of the country. Go to a different environment to test the child's condition. A dry environment or an ocean air environment is usually good for breathing problems. Consider an elimination testing diet program. Find a health care practitioner with experience in these skills.

The common food allergens or intolerances are: berries, buckwheat, chocolate, cinnamon, citrus fruits, corn (especially non organic corn), dairy products, eggs, mustard, any kind of nut, peanuts, peanut butter, pork, shellfish, soy, sugar, tomatoes, wheat and yeast. Also breathing in allergens from pets, animals, pollens, dust, chemicals or any other source including cleaners, lotions and soaps can cause adverse reactions. I would try to strengthen the body, if possible, rather than use pharmaceuticals for long-term treatment. I have known of several people who used inhalers for allergies all their lives and died during allergy attacks. I myself had pollen allergies as a child and luckily, I grew out of them and never used medications. If the body adapts to medication use then it may never be safe without it. Consult with a naturopath doctor.

In testing, you can eliminate suspected causes of adverse reactions one at a time, waiting a week or so for each to see how you feel. However, if you are getting bad reactions from multiple items, it will be difficult to feel a positive effect. For instance, if you have an allergic reaction to milk and wheat and if you drop the milk for a week and increase eating bread, you may not feel much better. I suggest eliminating all the common allergen foods that you suspect for a week or two, and then slowly bring them back one by one to see how you feel. Often people crave what they are allergic to, so do not be surprised if you crave something after you eliminate it. You may feel a little worse for a couple of days at first, do not give up. Wait the full period to judge how it is working.

Personally, I find it is difficult to tell a wheat allergy. I do think I have a very slight allergy to wheat, but it is so slight that I hardly feel it. However, if I stop eating wheat, I have an old knee injury that is slightly arthritic which gets better after a couple of weeks. In addition, my old foot injury gets dramatically better. I notice if I eat a large white wheat spaghetti meal or something similar with a lot of wheat or gluten, I get a bad feeling in my stomach. It feels like I am trying to digest a bowling ball! I can eat a little toasted bread fine at times, but overall my health is better when I eliminate processed wheat and gluten products.

Even with years of experience in self-monitoring my body, I still find it difficult to feel a slight negative effect to some food items. Like most people, I drank milk and ate wheat all of my early life. Even though we may not have had acute bad reactions in youth, some foods we thought fine might affect us negatively in older years. Sometimes it is a case of being fed what is considered good food by our parents, then later on realizing we always had a mild to acute negative reaction to something and did not know it.

Here is a short list of food items safe to eat for most people. Apples, apricots, asparagus, avocados, barley, beets, rice, broccoli, carrots, cauliflower, chicken, oats cranberries, dates, grapes, honey, lamb, lettuce, mangoes, papayas, peaches, pears, poi, raisins, rice, rye, safflower oil, olive oil, salmon, squash, sunflower oil, sweet potatoes, turkey and veal.

Of this list, I am personally allergic to beets, so it is possible to be allergic to something that is not a common allergen food. My wife is allergic to white potatoes, also not a common allergen food. I did not know I had an allergic reaction to beets until my thirties and my wife did not know she is allergic to white potatoes (Lectin allergy) until her forties. I know from experience, that people can have an on going negative reaction to a food or something else for many years and not know it.

All those nagging health problems, like asthma or joint pain and anything else that is bad and chronic. Any of these may be due to food intolerances, food allergens or parasites and you not know it. People can shrug these off for decades and keep on going, but as they get older, health problems become more severe.

Chapter Thirty Two

Fasting programs

Fasting is an old Biblical way to be healthier and to be closer to God. To fast you drink plenty of liquid and eat no solid food and this causes toxins to be released from the body. The body is designed to clean toxins out of fat and organs during times of famine. The longer the fast, the more toxins you remove. It is possible to go too far and starve, but few will do so. When we eat, breathe and are around chemicals, we take in toxins. These will build up inside the body. Some alternative health care providers estimate some people carry up to a pound of chemical toxins inside their body. These are accumulated over a lifetime.

The body tries to remove toxins in an ongoing basis, but often it cannot remove them all. Therefore, the body stores them somewhere, often inside the fatty tissue in and around body organs. If these toxins build up, serious illness can happen. I figure most everyone has stored up toxins needing to be cleaned out. Common medical care has few methods to remove these toxins. However, you can do so by fasting; all you need is the desire to be healthier.

The human body is designed to remove chemical toxins during times of fasting. Even in ancient times, there were toxins because some natural plants and food sources are toxic. In today's modern world a short period of forced fasting rarely happens, so cleansing never occurs.

During normal life, especially in today's toxin laden world it is inevitable that everyone will have toxins inside their body. If you have the desire and will power to fast, this is a way to remove these toxins. Removing toxins will help restore youth and vigor to your biological system. This is a real fountain of youth, not an imaginary one. Fasting in the correct way is a cleansing program to heal the body and to extend healthy lifespan.

Biblically, prayer and fasting is one of the most powerful ways to be closer to God. Almost all the saints and prophets fasted. Jesus and Moses both fasted for forty days. All the great figures in the Bible used fasts to communicate with God. A private non-boastful approach to fasting will lead you in being closer to God. Fasting and quiet prayer in a non-prideful way is the correct path. Real miracles can happen and the humble approach is the right method. Even whole communities of people can turn to fasting and prayer to seek help from God.

Why fasting works for health

By design, the body is very efficient at storing energy for times when no food is available. The body processes food in an expedient manner and is unable to remove all toxins in an ongoing basis. It must place immediate needs over the need to remove all ingested toxins in everyday life. For instance, in order for the body to remove all toxins in an ongoing basis could possibly mean twenty or more hours of sleep every day. This is impractical while living daily life. However, for many centuries forced fasting was a normal occurrence for people during famine, so cleansing happened then. Fasting in the past was sometimes by choice, but more often due to scarcity of food. The body would use this time for cleansing.

Even moderately thin people can go forty days without food. The body has a special mechanism to conserve energy and to clean toxins out of the body when food is limited. Fasting for health is not starvation, but rather a process of using stored energy while cleansing. Real starvation occurs when the body no longer has any stored energy and begins using organs for energy. Therapeutic fasts are ended before real starvation happens.

What happens during fasting?

For the first day or so, the body uses its glycogen reserves. These are energy-filled starches made and stored inside the liver and muscles of the body. After these are depleted, the body uses fat for energy. However, the brain, with its high fuel requirements needs glucose (sugar converted from glycogen) for energy. To obtain glucose sugar for the brain, the body begins to break down muscle tissue during the second day of the fast. Thus, during fasting, some muscle loss will occur, but this is fine. This is part of powerful cleansing and muscle mass may be recovered after the fast.

To fuel the brain, the body would need to burn over a pound of muscle a day, but the body has developed another way to create energy that saves muscle mass. This protein-sparing process is ketosis, which starts on the third day of a fast for men and the second day for women. The liver begins converting stored fat and other nonessential tissues into ketones, which are used by the brain, muscles, and heart for energy. Often the location of stored toxins is also the same place the body uses up nonessential tissues for energy during fasting. Therefore, the body removes toxins as it makes energy. Because the body is designed to use this muscle saving way of obtaining energy we know it is designed to handle fasting and to remove toxins while fasting.

It is at this point (2 to 3 days), in the fast that sensations of hunger go away for many people and some people experience normal or even increased energy levels. In addition, body functions become more stable after the first two or three days of the fast. The goal of water only fasting is to allow the body to reach the state of ketosis in order to burn excess fat and unneeded tissue, and remove toxins. Fasts that are longer than three days are generally the best therapy for health. Weight loss happens rapidly during the first few days of fasting, up to two pounds per day. In the following days, this number drops to around half a pound a day. An average weight loss of a pound a day for an entire fast may be expected.

The need for long-term water fast for deep

cleaning is rare. Less strenuous forms of fasting are also very beneficial. More common are maintenance fasts, such as the liquid nutrient fasts, or short-term water fasts. Long term fasting as a rule of thumb is longer than ten days, short term fasting is less than ten days.

Different types of fasts

Fasting is done different lengths of time depending on the person's desire and health condition. For chronic health problems, the strongest fast is two to four weeks of a water only fast, ending with broth or fruit juice during the last two to four days. Another kind of fast is a maintenance program fast, by fasting one day a week, or fasting three days ever so many months. A possible fasting program is a three-day fast every three months. It is convenient to mark the timing of these three-day fasts at the change of seasons.

Many people use liquid nutrient fasts or juice fasts. These are not strict fasts. Juice fasts are less powerful than water only fasts because the body does not reach the ketosis stage. Fruit and vegetable soup broth can supply energy, vital electrolytes and nutrition, which gently bathe the body in nutrients. Toxins are still removed, but not at the same intensity as a water only fast. Using a nutrient rich liquid allows fasting without a large drop in energy for working or doing other activities.

The disadvantage of liquid nutrient fasts is that the body never gets to the ketosis stage. It is thought by some to lack the deep detoxification of a water only fast. The advantage of a liquid nutrient fast is that it can supply some needed nutrition while still allowing detoxification. A more powerful water only fast can be done with distilled water. However, be careful, because distilled water will remove minerals along with toxins from the body. I would not do a distilled water fast long term. The danger is removing too many minerals from the body. This danger is even greater for those people who start the fast deficient; a nutritionally deficient condition is common for the sickly.

The danger is someone anemic in something, maybe anemic in iron, vitamins, and certain minerals. If so, a dangerous condition can develop when water fasting. It is best to seek professional medical help for any question. If you are in a fast and feeling really weak or faint, or having cramps, you should ingest liquid nutrition. The best is fresh organic vegetable soup broth with a little salt. Use fresh or dried organic vegetables when making this soup. These are full of minerals that can turn into electrolytes. In addition, you may consume fresh fruit juice or vegetable juice homemade with a juicer. In comparison, canned soup and pasteurized bottled juice is dead and deficient.

Medical supervision is best for any fast longer than three days *especially if the person is sickly*. Most alternative medicine practitioners, such as homeopaths and naturopathic doctors, can monitor patients during fasts. People performing extended fasts with health conditions may require blood, urine, and other testing during fasting. There are alternative health clinics that perform medically supervised fasts. Some conventional medical doctors may supervise patients during fasts and can help select the proper kind of fast. Fasting may be an alien concept to some professionals in conventional medicine, but it is as ancient and as accepted as the Bible. Find the right healthcare professional for your need.

Preparation for entering or leaving a fast

Fasts are better when you enter and exit them carefully. For preparation, it is best to eat a light diet with no meat, grains, nuts and processed foods for a day or two before starting the fast. The reason to have light foods before the fast is that there is nothing coming in to push food out. For instance, what is going to push out a giant beefsteak when you start fasting? Therefore, before a fast you want light foods that will go through the digestive system on their own, such as soft soups, light salads and fruits. This consideration is more important for extended fasting than short period fasting.

When ending an extended fast, start to drink any kind of liquid nutrient beforehand. Generally, you need two days time drinking liquid nutrients with soft foods before transitioning to solid food at the end of a long fast. Do not eat solid food when exiting a fast without a transition time using liquid foods, such as soup broth and juices. Your body is not ready for solid food; trust me it will hurt if you cheat.

When starting to eat solid foods choose something like soup with vegetables cooked to a soft mushy condition and soft fruit. Do not overeat, eat small meals and see how you feel. Wait until the second or third day before eating more solid foods. Do not have any tempting bad foods home when ending the fast.

Precautions and helpful activities during a fast

Fasters should drink plenty of fluid to move toxins out and to prevent dehydration. This means a gallon and more liquid a day, be mindful of your electrolyte and salt needs. Remember minerals from healthy live fresh food turns into electrolytes inside the body. A broth from vegetable soup with a little sea salt in it is great to obtain electrolytes. Saunas and sweating therapies may assist in detoxification, but must be used with good sense, if you are feeling faint and overheated then stop. It is helpful to walk, mow the grass, and work in the yard and garden. Any light exercise will move toxins out of the body.

A particularly helpful exercise is to bounce on a small trampoline. The body has a large circulatory system called the lymphatic system, which moves fat, white blood cells and lymph fluid around the body. It is helpful to stimulate it by exercising and therefore move toxins out of the body. The body's largest organ, the skin will emit toxins by sweating when exercising. It is good to bathe or shower two times a day to help remove toxins (use plain soap), and to scrape or brush the tongue. Enemas are good for health when needing intestinal colon detoxification-this improves the fast.

Side effects

People while fasting may experience side effects, such as fatigue, blurry vision, ill feeling, aches and pains, emotional duress, acne, smelly sweat, sweat with color, headache, swelling, bad breath, symptoms of colds and flu, and even vomiting. This happens because of the release of toxins from body fat and tissue into the circulatory system and going out of the body via the liver, kidneys, skin and other avenues.

I suggest for people who are chronically ill to not shock their body with a water only fast the first time fasting. It is better to do a short period liquid nutrient fast and later on consider longer fasts with either liquid nutrients or water. Some sources consider it healthier to fast with lemon water (or with some kind of juice depending on the desires of the faster) rather than water only fast. To make lemon water buy fresh lemons and a fruit squeezing bowl. Use at least half a lemon per quart of warm water. I like to eat a few lemon seeds (bitters) for better health.

If during a fast you are feeling extremely sick, consult with your health care provider about taking a few activated charcoal capsules to help remove toxins. This is an occasional treatment only when needed. Remember activated charcoal will absorb out medications. Alternatively, if feeling extremely weak in the legs start to drink clean fruit juice and vegetable soup broth to get electrolytes back up. If you feel mentally incoherent and have muscle cramps, then drink a soup broth with sea salt along with fruit juice. For people with diabetes or pre diabetic it is best to think about their body's response to fruit juices and fasting, and need help from a health care provider.

Depending on the stage of the fast, you can feel sickly, to really good or normal, then weak. Usually, you will feel hungry at first, and then somewhat normal, and later on get sickly, then again feel good, all these back and forth. After a longer period, you may feel weak. Often fasters cycle between feeling good, then sickly with headaches, back and forth, as waves of toxins are processing out of the body. Some ill feeling is normal, but if you are feeling like you are dying then consider taking activated charcoal or fruit juice or soup broth depending on symptoms. Once again, have medical care supervision. How bad a person feels depends on the initial health and weight of the person and how many toxins and parasites they have in their body and so on.

It is impossible for a book writer to know every possible human condition. Somewhat healthy people can handle sensible fasting fine. Sickly people may have serious problems and need professional monitoring. If you want to a do a fast with professional help, just look for the right kind of medical care provider with experience.

What to eat or drink during a fast

There are many ways to do a fast. The most common fasts are a water only fast, a fruit fast, a fruit juice fast, or any kind of liquid nutrient fast, even a light food fast. You can do almost any combination that you can imagine. For example, one may drink fruit juice, or some other kind of health drink or herbal drink for a specific health purpose. You can choose to fast by only eating light pulse foods and water.

As you can see there are many ways to fast, I once jokingly told my wife I wanted to go on a chocolate chip cookie fast! Seriously, one needs to think about the purpose of the fast. For most, it will be to become healthier. In order to achieve this goal you must feel hungry. That means fats and toxins are moving out of the body.

When fasting, the toxin-laden fats are in your blood stream, so you need plenty of liquid to get them out of the body. You will not feel good at times because there will be toxins moving out of the system. After about three days, many people start to feel better.

The length of the fast depends on the person and goals. Most will fast from one day to ten days. A forty-day fast is about as extreme as any should consider and most people should not fast for forty days. If doing a long term fast like forty days, it is best for most to drink fruit juice and maybe vegetable juice. Fruit juice puts carbohydrates into the system, which gives energy and still lets the body purge out toxins. If you decide to make vegetable soup, this will give the body electrolytes and nutrients. This soup has very little fat and protein, which helps the body get rid of toxins.

It is important for the body to eat proteins and fat from itself when fasting to get rid of toxins and diseases, such as cancer. To be hard-core in alternative treatment is to fast until the body must eat the cancer and diseased tissue for food. When toxin-laden fat is gone from around organs, the immune system can work better in that area of the body. It is good to have a parasite cleanse program before the fast.

Different plans for fasts

With guidance from your health care provider, here is a variety of various fasts to consider. For any of these fasts you can also drink herbal teas with different effects. Be very careful of strong herbal teas and seek expert advice. Herbal teas can help cleanse certain organs such as the kidneys or liver or remove parasites and other effects. I would be cautious of using any strong herb that you have no experience with during a fast, even with medical help. It may be better to test strong herbs before the fast to see how your body reacts. Below are fasting program ideas to consider.

1: Drink distilled water for three days, on the fourth day start drinking healthy fruit juice. Do this for three days. On the seventh and eighth day, eat fruit and a broth soup. Then start eating solid foods. If you eat solid foods too soon you will have stomach pains

2: Drink juices for five days, the last two days eat soft fruit. Then transition to a soft vegetable soup on the eighth day, and then slowly eat solid foods.

3: When ready, fast one day a week for a year. Eat fruit or drink fruit juice during the day and or distilled water.

4: When ready, fast two days a week for a year, best to do a liquid nutrient fast. Alternatively, have one day of distilled water and the second day with fruit juice, fruit, or a liquid nutrient drink.

5: Fast three to ten days every year, right after the new year is a good time. Drink lemon water and vegetable juices from homemade soup broths while fasting.

For any true fasting program, the main idea is to restrict unhealthy items and to eliminate out of diet, fats, proteins, and most carbohydrates. When the body is hungry for fats and proteins, it must take these out of the body for food, at the same time removing toxins. Any fasting variation should have this goal in mind to be effective.

Daniel's ten day fasting challenge

During the day, drink only apple juice and lemon water for ten days. Eat a light broth soup in the evening, while taking herbs for a parasite cleanse. Use fresh lemons and squeeze one-half to a whole lemon into each quart of warm water. Drink lemon water then flash pasteurized or fresh apple juice, alternatively all day long. Drink one glass of apple juice, then one glass of lemon water. You may use distilled water to make the lemon water more effective. Make sure you drink at least a gallon of liquid during the day. Force yourself if you must, this is important to get out the toxins.

Make fresh vegetable soup for the evening,

you can drink as much as you want. It will be broth and soft vegetables, lots of broth, eat the soup at a single setting. No oil in the soup and very little salt.

On the 11th day, start eating soft fruits and slightly more solid soup. The succeeding days start eating fats, proteins, and more solid foods.

Daniel's ten-day basic food fasting challenge

Eat only two meals a day. You can eat any food you want except no meat and unhealthy foods. It is a strict two meals only, with no snacking. This is not really a fast as you can live forever on this diet. It is a diet for most people because it is a restriction of food intake.

Most people snack at any twinge of hunger. If you cannot stop snacking, concentrate on eating only low fat and low protein alternatives, such as raw fruit and vegetables. Tomorrow is another day and eating raw foods during snacking is not a failure. You are still on a health program.

When you snack, is it because of true hunger or is it because of a stress reaction or a bad habit? It is best to have only healthy foods around when you get a snack attack. It is better to snack healthily than fight futilely against it, then give up totally. Have only healthy snack foods at home and in the car. It is fine to have an apple mid-day, especially when stressed. For ten days try to end all snacking and see how many days you can make it.

Daniel's super cleansing ten day fasting challenge

Buy an enema kit from the local drug store and have an enema the first couple of days during the fast. Drink only water and herbal teas for five to seven days. On days, nine and ten start eating soft fruits and mushy vegetable soup. On day eleven, break the fast with more solid foods.

Daniel's gentle 21 day fast for healing sickly people

This fast is based from my experience at a health retreat, where health experts were on hand. First thing in the morning take an herbal to get rid of parasites. Do this once a day for a few days. There are various ways and herbs to do this treatment. One way is one or two droppers full of tincture made of cloves, wormwood, and black walnut hull in a bit of warm water. I would suggest doing this parasite treatment for only about a week for most people. There are visual microscope tests to determine how toxic the blood is with tiny parasites. If these are present, then you need special attention from the correct medical care provider.

Have lemon water made from fresh real lemons, one or two lemons per quart of water every day. In addition, drink fresh made apple juice, or if this is too much trouble buy flash pasteurized apple juice or real cider.

The retreat used raw honey in the lemon juice to make it less sour. You can do this or have your lemon juice diluted with warm water.

All day long drink the lemon water and apple juice alternatively; one glass of lemon water, then one glass of apple juice. Most people do not drink enough liquid, drink a gallon and more. During the day walk and do light exercising. In the evening, have fresh vegetable soup broth made with a little sea salt. You also can eat some tomatoes and avocados if you like.

Mentally relax as much as possible, no negative influences, no news on TV, and no negative people. Watch comedies on TV and read light relaxing books. You will feel hungry and have energy, then no energy and feeling sick, then feel great. This happens alternatively and variably depending on the person and the stage of fast. If you are serious about health, think of doing enemas. How many and how often depends on how sick you are and your illness.

If you have constipation or bowel problems, you likely will need more enemas, but if no bowel problems then fewer enemas. It is possible to have stuck feces in your bowel that needs flushing and it may take several enemas. The majority of people only need a few enemas, one or two over the first two or three days until the bowel system is clean.

At day 21, you can start to take in soft protein and fat. Slowly eat more solid foods over a period of two days. This program is aimed to be as gentle as possible to remove toxins from the body. Nutritionally you are ingesting carbohydrates and liquids to flush out the fat toxins. In addition, you ingest electrolytes and nutrition from the soup-these will help cure deficiencies. To have strong detoxification, a fasting program should have no fat and protein intake.

After this fast, you are on the road of recovery. However, most extremely ill people need more fasting, careful diet, emotional rest, moderate exercise and a lifetime of positive lifestyle change. You should seek out the correct medical care practitioner to decide on your exact fasting program and to monitor condition.

For extreme long-term fasts with water or fruit juice, it is extra important to get help from a medical health care provider, especially for fasts longer than ten days.

A possible fast for healing is a water only fast until you get hungry again. I think hunger feelings differ from person to person. It is common that after day three of fasting hunger goes away and does not return until cleansed. This could be anywhere from ten days to thirty days and longer. This information is from my reading of some accounts of personal experience. If you eat or drink any nutrition during a fast, hunger never goes away as it does with pure water fast.

When ending a fast you will be extra hungry for fats and proteins. Find the cleanest sources of these to keep health.

If you do research, there are programs for cleansing different organs, such as watermelon to cleanse the liver and kidneys. If your liver or kidneys are aching, buy a whole watermelon and eat it. It should bring some relief in a few hours. Like any fruit fast, you can eat watermelon for a few days for more effect.

There are many ways to be closer to God. One way is to fast and walk with God in nature. While fasting, spend time outdoors, walking, fishing, mediating, biking, anything that is quiet and peaceful, even sun bathing while swimming. Have God on your mind and he will be with you.

When interacting with God, a common way is to plead and beg God. To ask questions, to ask for things, and ask for guidance. This is normal human nature. Another way is to just "be" and try to explore in a gentle way. God gave us free will, and he is likely interested in what we want to do in life-if it is positive. Answers to prayer may not be what we want them to be, lessons and blessings often come together in unexpected ways...

More about fasting cures for illness

A person may eat only one fruit for forty days and it may cure cancer. A person can select almost any favorite fruit, and then stick with it for forty days. My wife knew a man who had a tumor in his stomach years ago. He had little money and no health care insurance. Therefore, he went to an alternative health care provider who told him to select a single fruit and eat it for forty days and nothing else.

He selected grapes, and that is all he ate for forty days and he worked construction. During the last part of the fasting, he said it felt like his body was eating the tumor for food. After forty-days, the cancer was gone from his body. Then he ate normally and lived to be an old man.

However, he did drink grape juice every day for the rest of his life.

I think the cure worked because the fruit and water diet for forty days is an extreme cleansing program. In addition, since the body is not getting any fat or protein, it is in an extreme state of starvation for this nutrition. In the end, the body "ate" the cancer tumor for fat and protein. Understand the importance in following a correct program strictly. It takes an extreme state of hunger and cleansing until the body is able to devour cancer. I would not attempt such a fast without help from a health care provider to monitor physical condition. However, many conventional health care providers are negative about fasting treatments. If you want professional help in fasting, you will have to seek it out.

I think it important to go the full forty days, but longer may be harmful. Of course, after the fasting program you need to have the best diet and lifestyle possible. There are many kinds of fasting programs for illnesses and cancer. I would be cautious of a program with any new foods, especially exotic to you foods, avoid this. I would be cautious when using herbal treatments while fasting, strong herbs can be dangerous.

It is best to have medical testing afterward to see if the fast actually worked to remove the cancer or illness. If not, other treatments can still be done. What treatment chosen for illness is a personal choice. I have seen people die after conventional cancer treatments and after alternative cancer treatments. I have heard of and seen success after both kinds of treatments. A person with cancer should take in all information and do what is emotionally comfortable for them. If you chose conventional treatment, it is best to have the best diet and low stress lifestyle possible to help the treatment along.

I have been to a health retreat where there are many people with cancer. Most of them have terminal cancer. All went through the cleansing program for better health. The facility can only operate as a health improvement retreat. They do not diagnose or treat specific illnesses. It is only a general health improvement program. The liquid fasting program runs three weeks on, then a week off.

A person has special herbal teas in the morning, then glasses of lemon juice in water and apple juice alternatively one after another- the whole day, and a light soup meal in the evening. The people are to relax and take many walks during the day, and there are health lectures they can attend. The people get special herbal teas to remove parasites, to cleanse kidneys and liver, each in turn, one week at a time.

The people are not to eat any protein during the fast, even excess plant protein is restricted. It is so strict that they do not allow broccoli, because it has too much protein. The reasoning is even a speck of protein can allow cancer to continue to grow. Many people are there only after conventional medical care sends them home to die, or is unable to help them with various kinds of chronic illnesses. Most people go there to be healthier and a few go as their first choice for a health condition. Most are helped at least some. A few become well. Others have little to no success because they are too far along in illness.

The success rate is fair; I do not know the exact numbers of success verses failure. I think many people fail because they cannot keep up a good diet program after they go home. It is difficult to change lifestyle to a strict healthy one and rest and take it easy when away from the retreat.

Given that many people are terminally ill, the fasting program even with limited success gives people hope. Most people after fasting feel better for a time even if they do not fully recover. An ill person who goes to a good health retreat has a real chance of recovery. It is better to go sooner than later in my opinion. Another option is a mixture of treatments, some conventional and some alternative, and there are medical centers that offer this as well.

Chemical and radiation treatments will kill the cancer, but are also killing the patient and their immune system. It is a delicate balance, especially in extreme cases, to kill the cancer and not the patient. Even if most of the cancer is destroyed, a bit of cancer can explode into tumors in a short amount of time because of a weakened immune system. Thus, new treatment cycles may continue repeatedly until the cancer or the patient, or both are dead. If a person goes to an alternative fasting program after chemical treatments, it will be harder to build up the immune system. It may be better to use a fasting cleansing program as a first choice rather than a last resort. It is a personal choice, do your own research.

Any treatment program is not 100% certain of success. All can succeed or fail. Most alternative fasting treatments depend on having no protein or fat in the diet to help the body get rid of disease. Of course, the body needs protein and fat, so fasting cannot be kept up forever, but it must be long enough. Afterward, because of cleansing and parasite removal and nutrition, the body's immune system will start to work better. Conventional medicine can be used for diagnosis of diseases. The conventional treatment specialist will tell you the percentage of success of conventional treatment. Force them to define "success" as it may mean only some years free from cancer.

After research, you can think of what to do. Start conventional treatment or look for alternatives, one before the other or a mixture. If the conventional treatment has a high rate of real success, great, but also consider diet and lifestyle. In reality, it is far better to prevent illness by good health practices than making frantic efforts after serious illness. Have the best daily lifestyle for health because just one mistake may defeat all other efforts.

Beware, not all cleansing, fasting, alternative and conventional programs are equal. There are bad options out there. The best thing to do is talk to people who went through a certain program or are going through the program. No matter if conventional or alternative, take some time to do personal research. If you have no money for conventional treatment and no healthcare insurance, do not despair. Ask God for help and look for good books and inexpensive professional alternative healthcare people for help. With God, willpower, and desire, you have as good as chance as anyone, likely better.

It is a common mistake after a fasting treatment for a person when they feel better, (which commonly happens after cleansing programs), to try to do too much and go right back into a stressful lifestyle and eating bad foods. Usually this leads to health failure and right back into terminal illness, which is very sad. It is important to stick with the health program, to be restful and be in a low stress environment, *for the rest of your life.*

My first fast

My wife and I went on a fast together. She has been after me for years to do so. I was not mentally ready for a long time because it is an alien concept. I read some fasting books and was having slight headaches for over a week and steady kidney pain. Therefore, I was ready to go for it. Upton Sinclair's book "The fasting cure" is a great motivator in the health benefits of a fast.

The first three days are the hardest in terms of hunger. My personal experience and my wife's is you have bouts of weakness and faintness that pass in time. We were attempting a water only fast, but since we are doing this fast at the beginning of September of 2011, we had ripe blackberries on our daily walk. This was a too great of a temptation, so we ate these until full which is not that many since you get tired of them quick.

On day four, my wife convinced me that an enema is not that big of a deal. The mental barrier against the first enema is strong, but once achieved it is not so bad.   Therefore, we did enemas on day four and five. On the night of day four, we decided to eat a little vegetable soup broth, which helped my wife get past a tough point. I was having a slight amount of kidney pain on the morning of day five, after the enema this went away. I am happy with this personal discovery, as it shows me the possible benefit of an enema treatment for a health problem.

On day five, we decided to move toward more liquid nutrients. We ate a broth filled homemade vegetable soup. However, I was naughty, and ate some ice cream that night. Soon after my liver started to swell and I had diarrhea. I then took four activated charcoal capsules and threw away the rest of the ice cream. It tastes good and is so bad. It is best to have nothing of that sort in the house during a fast.

The next day I felt better overall. I still had touches of kidney pain, but about half or less than before the fast. The slight headaches I had the week before are gone. The next five days we drank apple juice, teas, store bought health drinks, and homemade vegetable soup. Our bellies were sensitive to solid foods at first and the softer foods were much easier. During the fast, I urinated a light brown colored pee, so I know I was detoxifying. In addition, during the last part of the fast, my wife and I experienced slight blurry vision. This indicates toxins are moving out of the body. Our vision cleared up once we started eating.

We both lost weight, about five pounds. Of course fasting is not a long-term plan to lose weight, but it is a side effect of cleansing.

Taking an Enema

This is how an enema works. There could be impacted feces on the walls of your intestines and in the colon, stuck there for who knows how long?   In addition, a person may have toxic matter stuck inside their intestines due to constipation. An enema can bring relief.   Matter stuck on intestine walls prevents the absorption of nutrients. The amount there depends on what you ate over the years and your ability to digest foods and genetics is a factor. I think most people would benefit from an enema every now and then. A good time to do one is during a fast. An enema may not remove all stuck matter, but it should remove some if not most. There are also herbal and pharmaceutical oral treatments that will remove stuck matter from intestines.

The way of the enema is not very noble, but it works for health. Buy an enema kit from the drug store. It is made up of a rubber bladder and a tube with an insertion end. It also has a valve that you hand operate to control the water flow. Fill the bladder with warm water, and hang it up on a towel rack in the bathroom. It has a hook made for to do this. Practice using the hand operated water valve by letting the water start and stop into the sink.

Lube up the insertion end of the enema

with petroleum jelly. Put down a towel on the bathroom floor, get down on all fours and insert end of enema tube into anus. Not fun, but it gets better as you get more petroleum jelly in around there. Then using the valve, you slowly fill up the colon cavity, if you put your butt up high and head down low this tends to get the water up higher in the intestines. This is a high enema. Using the control valve on the enema tube, you fill and stop filling as you slowly fill up the colon/intestines with water, as pressure builds up stop the flow, then start again when ready. Take in as much water as you can, when you feel like you cannot take anymore, then get on the commode. Sit for a few seconds and hold for a while, then relax and let go the water. You need to sit for a time as the water can be inside intestinal pockets and may come out unrepentantly if you get up too soon.

Keep repeating the process until all the water is gone from a single full enema bag. The last go around you need to sit on the commode for about five minutes to make sure all the water is gone. It is possible to empty the whole enema bag the first time or it may take several rounds. If you have toxic feces stuck in intestines and colon walls, this is what you need to get health back. If you are sick and have any toxic food inside your intestines, it will give great relief. These toxins, if left there, will continue to poison the liver, kidneys and whole body.

Once upon a time, the wife and I had an increase in funds after a period of lesser personal wealth. Therefore, we went to a couple of restaurants over the weekend and had a great time. However, the last eatery, which had great quantities of food, was a little too rich. The next morning I felt a little hung over in my mind and body, but otherwise fine. Unfortunately, my wife had a very painful back spasm attack during the day. She never had such attack before in her life! She had to lie down and take a couple of painkillers because the pain was so intense.

When learning her condition, I instantly started my mental motor thinking about her illness. I worked my mind trying to think of possible causes, can it be a lack of something such as lack of salt, minerals or maybe a female hormone change or because of food, we ate the night before? After she came to me, she drank some salt water and took some activated charcoal capsules. But, she had no relief from the spasms all that day and into the night. I tried to get her to take an enema that night, but she refused to believe it was the food because of no stomach or intestinal pains.

That morning I finally talked her into an enema and she did so, instantly she felt relief from half the pain. However, not from all the pain, I tried to talk her into a second enema, but she still did not want to believe the food was causing the back spasms. Also, she thought everything was out by the first enema. Therefore, no more enemas, but in a few days, all her back spasms went away....

The enema if done occasionally and carefully is an effective inexpensive at home treatment. Drug stores sell enema kits over the counter. Therefore, they are for consumer use as needed. I am surprised that activated charcoal capsules had little curative effect in this instance. The intestines needed an enema. (June 2012)

Recipe for vegetable soup and broth for fasting

Select an assortment of vegetables you are not allergic to, such as seaweed, cabbage, swiss chard, spinach, tomatoes, onion, broccoli florets (avoid broccoli if you have cancer, it has too much protein), summer squash, garlic, deacon radish etc. They can be any vegetable mixture that is soft when cooked. It is best to drink only the broth for hard-core fasting, but you may eat the soft vegetables if you want. Add a bit of sea salt while cooking. You could add in nutritional yeast for flavor and nutrition, but would detoxify better without it. Normally you add oil into soup, but for fasting, eating fats are counter productive.

That is it. Drink the warm broth, put leftovers in the fridge, use up leftovers and make fresh when needed.

The basic idea is obtaining nutrition while not defeating the purpose of the fast. Any clean liquid ingested gives the body what it needs to push the toxins out as the body feeds on its own fat and protein. The soup is for electrolytes and nutrients, the same for fruit or fruit juices. For fasting, the body must be hungry for fats and proteins, so only ingest clean foods that help the body eliminate toxins.

Two meals a day, is a daily fasting program

I went on an October 2011 trip to West

Virginia to see my folks, and go on a fishing trip to North Carolina on the ocean. We went camping and boating. I had a lot of fun and ate many garbage foods, and did not keep two meals a day. I have a family history of heart disease that I control effectively with diet and exercise. Nevertheless, I slip up at times, and the older I am the more I pay for it.

I suspect as I age in these modern times there are more and more additives and genetically engineered foods in the food supply. There can be additives that are below the 1% level, and not required by law to be on the food label. When I got back home to WA State, I had mild daily chest pains; for me this indicates a clogging of the heart and arteries.

While I was visiting in WVA a schoolmate, the same age as me (mid forties), died of a massive heart attack. A sad time and he had a new baby on the way. He had chronic chest pains for a long time. A warning that a heart attack is coming. The action that he could have taken in such a situation was to strenuously clean up diet. That means no processed foods, restricting saturated animal fats, and deep fried foods. For most people relief will be found by a strict health diet in a few weeks to a month or two. If not, fasting is needed or the conventional option is a bypass. Personally, I would choose fasting over the knife if I could. It is a choice. If you wait until a heart attack then it is likely too late to avoid surgery. If you have no access to expensive healthcare go on a strict health diet, the sooner the better and consider fasting.

Care must be taken when toxin-laden fats

are released into the system, especially in the beginning of a health diet program. If losing weight you may need to eat good fats to pace out the toxic fats going into the circulatory system from body fat. It is best for a health novice to seek out expert advice in diet and lifestyle, especially if sickly. The best diet lifestyle program must be followed for the rest of life. Most people will not change their lifestyle, so their only option is drugs and surgery. After a major heart attack, it is likely too late so you must have drugs and surgery to some extent. After a heart attack, chest pains may never go away, because of the physical damage.

I cannot know every chest pain situation. Some people may have physiological problems. However, in my own personal experience, if one will clean up the diet, it will clean out the arteries and veins to avoid heart attack. Most people are heading toward heart attack because of a diet that clogs up the system. Clean up the diet and get the crud out, then the odds of heart attack will drop down close to zero for most people.

I know of many people who think they eat healthy, but in my opinion, they are not doing well enough. Choose to believe you are eating healthy and not, you will pay for it. How can you tell if your diet is good enough? Here is my personal rough guide. If the new diet does not start to reduce chest pains in a week to a month, then it is not good enough. The right diet (with fasting for advanced cases, especially when older than forty) should reduce heart chest pains close to zero in a month or two. If not, something else is wrong other than clogged arteries or the diet is not good enough.

If you can afford it, get professional help and testing to know the exact cause of chest pain and to monitor progress with diet. Otherwise, use how you feel as a guide. There are tiny feeder arteries to the heart; if they are clogged, the heart is starved for nutrients and oxygen. Chest X-rays or other scans will show their condition, if clogged or not. This may be the source of chest pain, if so, clean out the crud and the pain should go away. It is that simple. If you wait until after a heart attack to take action, it is unlikely you will get health back. Many people do not survive their first major heart attack and have no second chance. Strong people even if thin may have clogged feeder arteries around the heart that can cause fatal heart attacks. Being relativity thin does not mean you do not have clogged arteries.

For myself I never had any health insurance, so I took personal action in diet and lifestyle, from chest pains to no chest pains *when I am eating correctly*. I do not favor drugs or surgery to clean out my arteries. I prefer improved diet and fasting. However, I do consider diagnosis by conventional medicine a good idea. In addition, if I could not control my diet then conventional treatments are the only option. Frankly, in my experience the vast majority of people would rather die than improve diet and lifestyle enough. Therefore, for most people drugs and knife cutting are the only option, because halfhearted attempts in better diet will not work. In my experience, it takes an extreme program in diet, fasting and exercise, to get health back. While only a semi good health program can maintain health.

So when I got back home I went to my strict two meals a day program that I had let slip up. After my evening meal I had no other food except a spoon full or two of lecithin in the late evening. Lecithin helps put any fat into solution in the blood stream. After a couple of weeks, I could feel my heart and arteries clean up because my mild chest pains went away. Most times a clean diet is enough for me. Rarely do I need a fasting program. In eating two meals a day, I have a daily fast after the last evening meal until the morning. If I ever feel the need for extra cleaning, I would do an extended fast.

For me, it is best to have some kind of regular fasting program all the time. I eat two meals a day, which is a kind of daily fast. This need is greater now for me than even a few years ago, because my metabolism is slower due to aging.

A particular problem for heart health is family social life. Most people even close friends and family will not understand your need for a strict diet. They may have bad foods, snacks, and drinks that are not healthy around you and get upset if you do not eat. A little will not hurt you, right? Oh yes it can. Do the best you can to limit bad foods while keeping a happy social life.

Chapter Thirty Three

An introduction to food additives and altered foods

There is an overwhelming list of over 3,000 food additives used in foods. They vary in effect concerning health. They are to improve on Mother Nature, to preserve food, make better texture or have something sweeter, creamier and more filling. Other than natural items, such as sea salt, or vitamins such as ascorbic acid, I figure most food additives are not good for human consumption. Of course, the possible exception is added vitamins and nutrients for fortification, which may have unfamiliar chemical sounding names.

In general, if you read a chemical name on a food label and not recognize it, you should look it up and see if it is a vitamin or something else healthy. Most often, food additives with unfamiliar names are not good for consumption. The more natural and original you buy food and prepare it fresh yourself, the healthier you will be. If you eat processed foods, additives may add up to many ounces of toxin ingested every year. The effect in your body may be slight or acute, depending on the amount and genetics. A person can be allergic to one or more of these additives and not know it. Since the amount of an additive in food may be a trace, it may be hard to feel a direct cause and effect while eating it.

On food product labels, additives may not be listed as ingredients when they are below 1% in concentration, depending on a particular nation's laws. This means any non-banned additive may be in any processed food or beverage and if below 1% not be on the label. Looking at items on product labels, the highest amount by weight is listed first on down the line. Therefore, the last ingredient or additive is the least amount by weight percentage. When eating processed foods, additives are the chemicals that make these products be all they can be, in taste, texture and shelf life. They are needed for large scale processing and distribution. Not all additives are bad for you, because some are from natural ingredients.

In general, if you have chronic ill health or mental problems start cleaning up diet and checking all food additives, looking for cause and effect. It is best to eat processed foods only occasionally. I think most processed foods and beverages have ingredients in them that are questionable for health. We hope that additives are in small enough amounts so our health will not be affected over lifespan.

Additives are inside processed foods and human history with these is short. Therefore, select the healthiest processed foods that you can find. However, it is better to make fresh food yourself from healthy source ingredients.

Example, I heard a story about a boy who drank excessively a certain citrus sport drink. I will not name the brand, but it is well known, and he drank it every day like water. After about a year of this, he started to gain weight and feel sickly. It turns out the manufacturers use bromide to extract citrus flavor out of lemons and limes. This bromide is in the sports drink so was building up inside his body. Once the boy stopped drinking the citrus drink, he got his health back. The lesson I got out of this example is that citrus drinks or any other processed beverage is acceptable only on occasion. To me this means once or twice a week and less. For occasional social functions, having a processed beverage is acceptable.

List of types of food additives

Acids

Food acids are added to make flavors sharper, and act as preservatives and antioxidants. Common food acids are vinegar, citric acid, tartaric acid, malic acid, fumaric acid and lactic acid.

Acidity regulators

Acidity regulators are in use to change or control the acidity and alkalinity of foods.

Anticaking agents

Anticaking agents keep powders such as milk powder from caking or sticking together or with other items.

Antifoaming agents

Antifoaming agents reduce or prevent foaming in foods.

Antioxidants

Antioxidants act as preservatives by inhibiting the effects of oxygen in food. Oxygen will oxidize food to cause spoilage.

Bulking agents

Bulking agents such as starch are additives that increase bulk of a food inexpensively without affecting taste, for example, non-organic cornstarch in yogurt, which I must avoid.

Food coloring

Colorings are added to food to replace colors lost during processing, or to make food look more attractive. Some foods are unnaturally colored for display. However, people think it is natural because it is the familiar food color they see all their lives.

Color retention agents

In contrast to colorings, color retention agents are to keep existing color.

Emulsifiers

Emulsifiers allow water and oils to remain mixed together, for example in mayonnaise, ice cream, and homogenized milk.

Flavors

Flavors are additives that give food a particular taste or smell. These are derived from natural ingredients or created artificially.

Flavor enhancers

Flavor enhancers improve on existing flavors. They are extracted from natural sources; through distillation, solvent extraction, maceration, or even created artificially from chemicals.

Flour treatment agents

Flour treatment agents are added to flour to improve color or other qualities for baking.

Glazing agents

Glazing agents provide a shiny appearance or protective coating to foods. They are often sweet.

Humectants

Humectants prevent foods from drying out. They are moisturizing agents.

Tracer gas

Tracer gases are for testing package integrity, thus preventing foods from being exposed to air.

Preservatives

Preservatives prevent or inhibit spoilage of food due to mold, fungi, bacteria and other microorganisms. Most natural foods rot when left out for a few days. Foods with preservatives last much longer. For example, if you put a store bought candy bar outside, it will hardly rot. Naturally made bread will not last as long as store bought bread with preservatives. If a store bought food can be left out for many days with no mold or rot. It likely has unhealthy preservatives.

Stabilizers

Stabilizers, thickeners and gelling agents like agar or pectin give foods firmer texture. An example of use is in fruit preserves. They also help to stabilize emulsions.

Sweeteners

Sweeteners are added to foods for flavoring. Artificial sweeteners are in low calorie foods. Sugar is in everything and can be harmful to health in quantities consumed by most people. Most artificial sweeteners are harmful as well. It is best to limit all of these. Once you are used to natural foods, added sugar tastes too sweet.

Thickeners

Thickeners are substances when added to a mixture will increase viscosity.

As you can see from this list, processed foods have additives for many purposes, to improve taste, texture, smell and shelf life of a food or beverage. Additives may have negative health effects.

A partial list of altered foods and beverages and their effects

Refined grain products

In Biblical times, stone grinding processed wheat and other grains. This created a whole course grain for making food or bread. In modern times, steel processing machinery removes bran from wheat and grinds the grain up into very fine flour. Bran is the outside layer that is hard and has additional nutrients and fiber. This new fine flour without bran enables the production of nice smooth textured foods, breads and pastries. (One can buy the separated bran to put in food for additional nutrition.)

The problem with these new fine flours is

that people are not designed to eat them in quantity. High glycemic carbohydrates in excess such as from finely processed grains put an extra strain on the pancreas and body because they are quick to digest. Stay away from finely ground grains and look for more natural course grain products and breads, like stone ground wheat products or natural brown rice products. This is more important if you are overweight, with diabetes or have a family history of diabetes. If you do not have diabetes yet, avoiding fine flour products may help prevent the onset.

Salt

If you are eating many processed foods, it is possible your eating excess salt. Salt is important for health and life, and the more you exercise and sweat the more salt you need. It is possible to be on a health diet and not get enough salt. Therefore, do not go to an extreme either way. If you are muscle cramping feeling faint and craving salt, then you may need more salt. Alternatively, if you are suffering from high blood pressure and or kidney pain, you may have too much salt in the diet.

Taste your sweat. Body sweat should have a faint salty taste, not too strong or too weak. A person severely low in salt can be faint and weak or even go into shock. This usually happens when the person is hot, working hard and sweating. If in this condition, you may take a tiny pinch of sea salt with water or a sports drink with electrolytes. Note: too much salt eaten at once can dangerously shock the body, for example, a teaspoon or more of salt all at once can be dangerous. Carefully and slowly take in electrolytes and or salt with water until feeling better while not over doing it.

Salt intake is something that can fluctuate daily, so monitor it. People need a little salt every day, not zero salt and not an excessive amount of salt. A few shakes of the saltshaker into food while cooking should be correct for most people, depending on how much salt they intake from processed foods. Most people should have no more than 1/2 of a level teaspoon of additional salt in a day (over what is in their food), spread out over the whole day. The optimum can be less, maybe a 1/4 teaspoon in a day-down to zero if eating many processed foods with salt.

Sea salt verses ordinary table salt. Ordinary table salt usually has an anticlumping chemical in it and little natural trace minerals. Sea salt has trace minerals from the sea inside it. Table salt may have iodine added to it because society found that many people have iodine deficiency. This deficiency causes goiter and low IQ in children. I personally prefer sea salt with natural trace minerals in it, also added Iodine in sea salt is beneficial. Different sea salts have different amounts of minerals and colors. Shop around to find what you like best.

Iodine deficiency can lead to many chronic health problems and is common without supplementation. Iodine added to salt is typically a minimum to prevent thyroid goiter (an enlarged thyroid causing a lump at the throat). It is common to need iodine supplementation for optimum health. Goiter is an indicator of extreme

High fructose corn syrup

Food manufactures use cornstarch to make corn syrup. Remember corn is often a genetically modified crop. Industry adds enzymes to corn syrup and uses further processing to create a sweetener that is 55% fructose and 45% sucrose. This product and variations are inside many processed foods. The biggest danger is not the sweetener, it is the quantity eaten.

Before modern production methods, the only sweets in foods came from natural sources, and these sources depended on the season. The human body does not have a genetic background to allow large amounts of sweeteners in the diet. For instance before modern times, if we assume the average consumption of natural sweeteners was about 8 grams a day, that adds up to about 6.5lbs per year. The average yearly intake of high fructose corn syrup in the USA is 38lbs in 2008. This is a multiple of about six times over ancient human history for this one sweetener alone.

I often have an adverse reaction from corn products; I get a headache and generally feel bad. This lasts for a day to several days depending on how much I ate. This started for me around 2004. I suspect it is because of genetic modification, I eat organic corn products with no ill affect.

Sugar from beets

Beet sugar is also a relatively new process first started in the 1800's. In 2005, extensive use of a certain genetically modified beet plant started because farmers could use a weed control agent with it. This enabled greater usage of mechanical means of production for more beet sugar. Of course, there is very little human history of eating beet sugar of any kind, especially beet sugar made from genetically modified plants. Today the average person consumes their body weight in sugar a year. The bulk of this consumption is divided up between sugar from beets and sugar cane. The average person in the USA consumes over 50 pounds of beet sugar and over 50 pounds of cane sugar in a year!

To avoid eating too much sugar is simple. Do not eat processed foods made with sugar.

Sugar from cane

Sugar cane has a long history and was grown as long as 5000 years ago. It was used for several centuries as a food in different regions of the world. Like other sources of sugar, modern day processing has changed the nature of sugar made from cane. As a general rule, all forms of sweetener from manmade products should be restricted for health. Remember that the average human body's genetics has no history with high amounts of sugary foods. The average body has no safe way to deal with excessive sugar and refined high glycemic index carbohydrates. It is easy to eat these in excess and not know it due to modern culture. No matter the source of sugar or refined carbohydrates, excess will destroy health.

One ongoing concern is the changing nature of food due to even newer processes and genetic engineering. New bad reactions to food can emerge for you even when eating familiar foods. A general rule for good health is choosing the most natural organic sweeteners that you can find. Choose natural brown cane sugar, raw honey, brown rice syrup for sweeteners and use little as possible.

A rule of thumb when cooking is to cut the sugar in recipes in half or even down to a quarter.

Artificial sweeteners

These are chemically made to replace sugars. Acesulfame-K, As-partame, Equal®, NutraSweet®, Sac-charin, Sweet'n Low®, Sucralose, Splenda® & Sorbitol). Some of these are linked to cancer; and they may cause an adverse reaction for sensitive people. Consider only using moderate amounts of natural sweeteners, or no sweetener at all.

Genetic Modified Organism (GMO) foods

There has been an explosion of genetic engineering since the mid 1990s. We are in a time of unknown foods and the outcome is uncertain. It is an ongoing experiment on the human population. A warning sign is the dying of honeybees living on modern farm crops. It is a struggle to protect ourselves from unforeseen effects of modern food production. It is important to buy organic as much as possible. In using genetically modified foods there is real time experimentation going on the human population. Only when enough people get sick, will industry be forced to change something back and or take it off the market. I wonder if there will be vast waves of forever-sick people, creating a health crisis. I consider this very likely. It is already the case with diabetes. Diabetes is mild as compared to what may happen.

When selecting meat I prefer free range meat, which means grass fed not grain fed animals. In health food stores, you can buy meat from animals raised without hormones and antibiotics, which is a step up, but they still fatten these animals with grain. I suggest buying free-range meats for better health. These are grass fed animals and are the superior animal protein. Grass fed animals have less fat and the meat quality is better. It is closer to what the human body has used throughout history, what the maker intended. Ancient man obtained some calcium and phosphorous from bone. Modern day people may use soup bones and eat clean fish with bones cooked inside. Canned salmon and sardines are two common sources today.

Food irradiation treatment

Food irradiation is a new development in the last hundred years; industry zaps food and containers with ionizing radiation. This changes the nature of the food and may create harmful chemicals or altered foods in trace amounts. The long-term effect of this process is unknown; this effect may be slight or great? If you buy organic you may avoid irradiated food. There is no requirement in the USA for labeling radiation treated food.

The items approved for irradiation in the USA are shellfish, wheat flour, white potatoes, pork, fruit, vegetables, spices, poultry, meat, yeast, enzymes, and poultry feed. Common on the market are irradiated herbs, herb teas, garlic, spices, and some ground beef, fruits, and vegetables.

Labeling of fresh fruits and vegetables

You can tell if foods are commercially or organically grown or GMO. Just look at the item itself, or on the pricing on the food stand, for a four or five digit number.

1. Four digits, it is conventionally grown.
2. Five digits, starting with the number 8, then genetically modified.
3. Five digits, starting with the number 9, then organic.

Pasteurization

In modern production pasteurization is very important for public safety, but not so good for personal health when compared to safe natural products. Most processed beverages are pasteurized, usually by heat. This destroys vitamins and enzymes and makes a live food into a dead one. The solution for this is to buy drinks that are made with the least amount of pasteurization and still safe. I like drinking flash pasteurized apple juice, which is a step up in health.

The best juice is homemade from fresh fruit, but many of us cannot afford this practice nor have the time. I go to the health food store and buy refrigerated health drinks made with a minimum amount of processing and kept cold to prevent spoilage. In addition, there are juicer restaurants where you can buy fresh made juice. Make it a daily habit to choose live safe foods, drinks and your health will improve.

Partially Hydrogenated oil

Partially hydrogenated oil may be labeled as hydrogenated oil, or fractionated oil. This oil can be very hard to digest by the human body. It is a preservative and prevents the natural decay of fatty foods. I like to think of it as turning the oil into a type of plastic. Some people can handle this altered oil better than others. For many people it is deadly because it will contribute to heart disease and heart attacks. My personal experience is that when I eat food with a lot of partially hydrogenated oil, I feel like my heart is pumping sludge through my arteries. I also have chest pains. I suggest staying away from hydrogenated oil, especially if you have a family history of heart disease.

Any store bought item that has a long shelf life is suspected to have preservatives inside it and/or altered oils that may be hard to digest and can build up sludge in your system. If you are having chest congestion or chest pains due to artery clogging, then change eating habits or you are going to have a heart attack. It is a good idea to have chest x-rays of the heart *before* the heart attack. It will give you a chance to clean up your diet, and to remove the sludge by fasting. There are other causes of chest pain rather than artery clogging, so it is best to be checked out by a doctor if you can. It is possible to be clogged up and not have clear-cut chest pains; this situation is more likely for women. Pay close attention to any strange pains in the arms, back or neck, especially for women.

There is an epidemic of USA men in the 30's to 40's+ having heart attacks and dying. I suggest watching the men in your life and getting them to change their eating patterns, especially if they are having chest pains. They may have ongoing chest pains for years and not say much of anything. See a heart specialist as soon as possible.

If a person will change their diet to a clean one using lecithin and hot peppers, the pains will go away in a matter of weeks to months for most people unless they are extremely unhealthy. If a person will not change their diet, they must take drugs and have surgery. However, with a clean diet, unless it is too late after a heart attack, many if not most people should not need drugs. By clean diet, I mean very clean. If you are having, chest pains due to artery clogging, you know your diet is not clean enough-it is that simple. A fast or several fasts may be necessary as well.

In my personal experience, if I get off a

clean diet too long, it takes one week to three weeks of clean eating for my chest pains to go away. My chest pains are due to eating too many processed goods, primarily regular store bought cookies. Much of this depends on genetics, I notice some people handle processed foods better than others do.   Remember, new preservatives and altered foods are coming on the market all the time, and if an additive is less than 1%, it may not be on the food label. Stay on your toes, trust nothing, read all food labels, use how you feel as the final guide.

I notice now in my mid forties that I need to think more about fasting to get the crud out of my system. As people get older, a fasting program is more likely to be needed. Consider a three to ten day juice fast once a year, especially if past the age of forty. Sooner, if you are having serious chronic chest pains before the age of forty. Same for any chronic illness that will not go away, consider fasting.

Food Coloring

Most food colorings are made from coal tar or synthetic coal tar. Others are derived from natural plant sources; these are at various levels for being healthy. Some of these food colorings have been banned; others are not and cause bad reactions for people such as hyperactivity in some children. Not all colorings are unhealthy since some are naturally made. Food coloring is added to give the consumer the comfortable feeling with a familiar color that they are used to. For instance, the brightly colored red meat you feel warm and fuzzy about when purchasing may be due to food coloring.

The USA FDA receives compensation for every pound of food dye it certifies (most dye is not inspected, only spot inspections); some see this as a conflict of interest in regard to the safety of these dyes. They are 100 Curcumin, turmeric; 101 Riboflavin -Vitamin B2; 102 Tartrazine; 103 Chrysoine Resorcinol; 104 Quinoline Yellow; 107 Yellow 2G;   110 Sunset Yellow FCF; 120 Cochineal, Carminic acid; 122 Carmoisine; 123 Amaranth; 124 Brilliant Scarlet 4R, Ponceau 4R; 127 Erythrosine; 128 Red 2G;   129 Allura Red AC; 131 Patent Blue V; 132 Indigo Carmine; 133 Brilliant Blue FCF;   140 Chlorophyll; 141 Copper complex of Chlorophyll; 150(A-D) Caramels; 151 Brilliant Black BN;   153 Carbon black, Vegetable carbon; 154 Brown FK; 155 Chocolate brown HT; 160(A) Alpha-, Beta-, Gamma-Carotene;   160(B) Annatto, bixin, norbixin; 160(C) Paprika extract, Capsanthin; 160(D) Lycopene;   160(E) Beta-apo-8'-carotenal; 160(F) Ethyl ester of beta-apo-8'-carotenic acid;   161 Xanthophylls;   161(G) Canthaxanthin; 162 Betanin (Beetroot Red); 163 Anthocyanins;   170 Calcium carbonate, Chalk; 171 Titanium dioxide;   172 Iron oxides and hydroxides;   173 Aluminium;   174 Silver;   175 Gold;   180 Pigment Rubine, Lithol Rubine; 181 Tannin, Tannic acid.

A partial list of preservatives

Sorbates

Sorbates are naturally inside fruit. When used as a preservative, they inhibit fungal growth, but allow for bacterial activity. They are obtained from the berries of mountain ash or synthesized from ketene. When used as a preservative in cosmetics and pharmaceuticals sorbates can be a skin irritant and may cause rashes, asthma and hyperactivity. They are in use in wine, cheese, fermented products, dessert sauces, fillings, soups, sweets, drinks and yeast goods. They are 200 Sorbic acid; 201 Sodium Sorbate; 202 Potassium Sorbate; 203 Calcium Sorbate.

Benzoic acid and its salts

Benzoic acid and its salts inhibit the growth of mold, yeast and bacteria. Its salts are created from reactions with sodium, potassium and calcium salt. These are in alcoholic beverages, baked goods, sugar substitutes, cosmetics, dried fruits, processed fish, pickled products, margarine, fruit sauces, and preserves.

Benzoic acid salts are inside products typically at .05% to .1% in concentration; anything less than 1% may not be on the food label in the USA. A similar situation is possible in other countries as well. This family of preservatives may cause contact skin reactions or other adverse reactions when ingested, such as asthma. They are 210 Benzoic Acid; 211 Sodium benzoate; 213 Calcium benzoate; 214 Ethyl para-hydroxybenzoate; 215 Sodium ethyl para-hydroxybenzoate; E216 Propylparaben;

E217 Sodium propyl para-hydroxybenzoate; 218 Methyl para-hydroxybenzoate; 219 Sodium methyl p-hydroxybenzoate.

Sulfites

Sulfites are among the top nine preservatives for adverse reactions. Asthmatics or people with known sensitivity to aspirin need to be extra cautious. They were banned in 1996 in the USA for use in fresh foods. They still are in use for beer (hang over), soft drinks, dried fruit, juices, cordials, wine, vinegar and potato products. Sulfites are known to cause gastric irritation, nausea, diarrhea, skin rash and asthma attacks. They are difficult to digest for people with impaired kidney function (may feel kidney pain), and sulfites destroy vitamin B1 (thiamin), and should be avoided by anyone suffering from conjunctivitis, bronchitis, emphysema, bronchial asthma and cardiovascular disease. They are 221 Sodium sulphite; 222 Sodium hydrogen sulphite; 223 Sodium metabisulphite; 224 Potassium metabisulphite; 225 Potassium sulphite; 226 Calcium sulphite; 227 Calcium hydrogen sulphite; 228 Potassium bisulphate.

Formic acid.

Formic acid is used as a preservative in food, the manufacturing of leather and in preparation of latex rubber. They are 236 Formic acid; 237 Sodium formate; 238 Calcium formate.

Formaldehyde

Formaldehyde is very toxic to breathe, to ingest and take in by skin absorption. Fumes are easy to breathe in and absorbed through the skin. It is a cancer hazard. Formaldehyde may cause damage to kidneys and can cause acute adverse reactions, such as sinus headaches. It is extremely destructive to mucous membranes, the upper respiratory tract and to the eyes and skin. It is used in industrial processes and sometimes-in foods and beverages legally and illegally in some countries. It is in bedding and building products, especially in new products made of foam or filled with glue.

Formaldehyde gas is more concentrated in new products and new construction. Watch out for children and sensitive people with new products emitting toxic fumes. A new product needs to age for a year or more to get much of the toxic gas out. It may be better to buy older products than new, or let new products age before usage. For example, I just obtained a ten-year-old foam mattress comforter and I am very happy with it, no toxic smell at all! A new foam comforter may have a slight smell and cause a headache for me. It is 240 Formaldehyde.

Nitrates

Nitrates and nitrites are chemicals that are naturally in our environment. Nitrogen and oxygen combine to form these nitrogen-containing compounds. Nitrates are essential nutrients for plants to grow. They are in the air, soil, surface water and in underground drinking water. Nitrates are in use for fertilizer and are naturally in decaying plant and animal matter. The environmental problems start when man made nitrites/nitrates go into the environment at a too great rate.

Excess nitrate concentrations get into surface water and in lakes, streams and bays. This happens mostly by surface run off from fertilizers and animal waste, such as manure from cattle and pig farms, from sewage plants and septic systems. Harmful human over exposure happens by eating meat preserved with nitrates and vegetables with excess nitrates in them (from chemical fertilizer) and from drinking contaminated well water in farming areas.

Vegetables account for more than 70% of the nitrates in a typical diet. Cauliflower, spinach, collard greens, broccoli, and root vegetables contain higher amounts of nitrates than other plant foods. About 6% of human exposure comes from meat products. Sodium nitrate in processed meat is in use as a preservative and color-enhancing agent. Most vegetables are not grown organically and are fertilized chemically with nitrates rather than with manure. Some nitrate ingestion is normal and healthy in the diet. The problems for people start with excessive concentrations inside the body.

Acute nitrate poisoning can deprive the body of oxygen and cause blue skin. This can be especially dangerous to infants. Ingestion of nitrates may cause hyperactivity in children and other adverse reactions. It may cause cancer after ingesting an excessive amount over time. They are linked to throat cancer, stomach cancer, colon cancer, prostate cancer and pancreatic cancer. To avoid excess nitrates in the diet eat organic vegetables as much as possible and avoid eating processed meats. Nitrates are 249 Potassium nitrite; 250 Sodium nitrite; 251 Sodium nitrate-saltpeter; 252 Potassium nitrate.

Acetates

Acetic acid or ethanoic acid has been used for hundreds of years as a natural preservative in vinegar. During the fermentation of grapes or other fruits, oxygen is allowed into the container. Then bacteria convert the ethanol into ethanoic acid causing the wine to sour into vinegar.

261 Potassium acetate is the potassium salt of acetate. It can be dangerous for people with kidney problems. 264 Ammonium acetate may cause nausea and vomiting. 262 Sodium acetate and anhydrous sodium diacetate have no known bad effects.

Propionates

Propionates may be linked to migraine headaches for some people. Propionates occur naturally in fermented foods, human perspiration and in the rumen part of the digestive tract of cud chewing animals.

Propionates are derived commercially, and commonly used in bread, cheese and flour products. They can cause irritability and other problems in children when eating products containing this additive, notably bread. Propionates are 281 Sodium propionate; 282 Calcium propionate; 283 Potassium propionate.

Boric acid

Used as a preservative and bleaching agent, boric acid is an antiseptic. It is also used in insecticides. A common use is to make lines of it around a kitchen or a room to kill cockroaches and ants. They pick it up on their feet when walking over it and ingest it when licking it off. In addition, one can make a bait of sugar, boric acid and flour in a pan. They will be attracted to the sugar, eat the boric acid and die.

Boric acid has many safe uses and it takes a relatively large amount of it to be lethal in a single dose. Nevertheless, as a food preservative it is harmful to kidneys and overall health. Used in soaps and many other industrial processes, it is toxic when ingested and may cause liver cancer, typically not used inside food except illegally in some Asian countries. Examples are 284 Boric acid; and 285 Sodium tetraborate (Borax).

Synthetic antioxidants

Gallates are used to prevent oily foods from spoiling. It is an antioxidant, which works by preventing oxygen from combining with oil and going rancid. It causes stomach discomfort and skin irritability and adverse reactions that affect the ability to breathe. It may cause kidney and liver problems. They are 310 Propyl Gallate; 311 Octyl gallate; 312 Dodecyl Gallate.

TBHQ, BHA, BHT

These are used to preserve oil, dairy, margarine, dressing, lipstick, chewing gum, and instant potato products. They are not permitted in infant products. They may cause hyperactivity with other adverse reactions and even cancer in high dosages. They were banned in Japan in 1958. They are 319 Butylhydroxinon; 320 Butylated Hydroxyanisole (BHA); 321 Butylated hydroxytoluene (BHT).

Flavor enhancers

Glutamates

These improve taste by giving a meaty salty flavor to foods. They are used in sauces or on foods for a sauce like coating. Glutamates are in over ten thousand foods in the USA!

Glutamates may kill nerve cells, resulting in nerve degenerative diseases such as Lou Gehrigs, Multiple Sclerosis, Huntington's, Alzheimer's and Parkinsons. Glutamates may cause trouble for asthmatics. They may be in canned foods, canned meat and vegetables.

Glutamates can cause nerve damage and should be avoided by children and infants. They may cause any kind of nerve disease. It is possible that as much as 30% of the population negatively reacts to MSG. To avoid eat only frozen, fresh or dried organic products. Glutamates are 620 L-Glutamic acid; 622 Monopotassium glutamate; 623 Calcium glutamate; 624 Mono ammonium glutamate; 625 Magnesium di glutamate;

Most of us do not think about harmful additives in our foods that are comforting and nourishing. However, let us take one example, bread. Biblically, bread is the source of life, but common commercial bread of today is nothing like Biblical bread. Biblical bread is made from a combination of course stone ground grains with nuts and seeds. Ancient bread is often so dense and heavy that it needs to be dipped in water, milk or oil to soften it so it can be chewed and swallowed. Today bread is made from super fine flour, which makes it high in the glycemic index. In addition, modern bread usually has additives to improve taste, texture and shelf life.

Consider avoiding breads for a week to a month and see how you feel. For instance, to see how your joints are doing without breads. For me, my knee joints feel better when I am avoiding modern breads. Gluten and additives in bread may be detrimental to your overall intestinal and joint health due to adverse reaction.

Epilog; Living by Biblical Daniel's example

Biblical Daniel made some predictions during his life with the king. The basic account goes like this. King Nebuchadnezzar had a nightmare and called in his wise men to interpret the dream, but *first he demanded for them to describe his dream to him!* Of course, they could not, therefore the angry king threatened to kill all the wise men! Daniel heard of this and being one of the men the king was going to kill, he was very afraid. Therefore, he prayed to God for help. In response, God gave Daniel a vision about the king's dream. Then Daniel went to the King. He told the king his dream and its meaning. Thus, the king spared everyone's life.

The king's dream predicted the end of Babylon and the end of all nations, leading up to the end of time on earth. As part of the dream, it was predicted that the great city-state Babylon would be destroyed and never exist again. In the ancient world, the city-state Babylon was most powerful. Nevertheless, Babylon was destroyed long ago and has never existed again. Pictures of the ancient ruins are in modern day Iraq. You can look them up on the internet.

In life no matter what time in history we live, there are difficulties. Biblical Daniel was taken from his homeland to live in a foreign land and made into a eunuch slave. As a slave he had to serve a foreign king with a different language, religion and lifestyle.

Biblical Daniel's example shows his strength of character in extreme adversity. His story has stood far longer than Babylon, the most powerful city-state in Daniel's time. It was an oppressive cruel nation without God's blessing, so it destroyed itself forever by its own actions.

Many people in all times have difficult lives similar to Biblical Daniel. Understanding Daniel's example, anyone can build a relationship with God and try to do what is right and God will help. Strive for a positive frugal lifestyle, choose friends carefully and tie into the community. In hard times, it is best to have some hobbies that help economically. Look for side businesses and second jobs rather than frivolous expensive hobbies. Daniel's example shows always to do good work, even the small tasks.

If times are good for you, let us say for seven years, save up for a possible seven years of famine as indicated in the Bible. Find your roots in faith and be self-sufficient as much as possible, know how to enjoy a simple life. Grow a garden, plant fruit trees, learn a trade and enjoy the simple things. Avoid excessive consumption. The wise person will build their house (and life) up high on rock, not down low on sand near water. He or she can live happily within a simple life doing productive work.

The Bible says God will protect his people in hard times. I believe any person of faith can be part of God's people; only God knows your heart. Strive to become the person you want to be, work well and be honest. Be slow to anger and quick to forgive. However, do not let others continuously abuse you or immoral people influence you. Moral and non-moral people are everywhere. Some people may use their version of Godly morality as a hammer on others and take advantages.

I find in life there are direct blessings from God. In addition, there are lessons that he teaches by life's trials, remember this as you pray and live. Often lessons are in combination with blessings from God. For example, you may pray for help and receive a mental impression to do something. This action may be emotionally or physically difficult to do, but beneficial. The impression should never be anything harmful or dangerous.

Many people pray for wealth, power or commercial things. God has much patience; however, it is rare that God will simply give things for a person's consumption. Think about what you are asking for. Think about the lessons you may need to learn. God may be trying to teach you something by your trials. He can teach for a lifetime and some people never learn their lessons. He knows your heart, your deceit, conceit, ego and sins.

I suggest following the Ten Commandments and reading the stories of the Bible as lessons for a better life. People who break the Ten Commandments are likely to suffer, and cause suffering. Paying tithe is a lesson many Christians cannot bear. One of the hardest tests for the faithful is to pay tithe with no pride, especially in lean times. Lessons and blessings, they will come to you if you try the path of communicating with God while asking for guidance. There is only one way to understand what this means, by developing a relationship with God.

I understand many people are not comfortable with organized religion. No matter you can privately develop a relationship with God. It is best to ask God for day-to-day help in moral character, for correct action and for real needs. Give thanks for what you have every day.

Not many people will follow Biblical Daniel's example in life. Most would rather saw off a limb than improve on what they eat and how they live. Few will eat plain pulse foods over tasty processed foods and give up addictive bad habits. Some good does not outweigh the bad in diet and lifestyle. If you pray and work toward following Biblical Daniel's example, you are one of a *few* and will benefit.

References

I used all of these health resources and more to create this book. Here is a list of health books that I think would be helpful to own.

"Prescription for Nutritional Healing" by Phyllis A. Balch, cnc. (Reference)

"The Natural Remedies Encyclopedia" by Vance Ferrell and Harold M. Cherne, MD. (Reference and to read)

"The cure for all Diseases" by Hulda Regehr Clark, Ph.D., ND. (Reference and to read)

"Back to Eden" by Jethro Kloss. (Reference and read)

"Left for Dead" by Dick Quinn. (Story and reference, to read about heart disease)

"The Makers Diet" by Jordan S. Rubin. (Story and reference)

"The Complete Book of Minerals for Health" By Sharon Faelten.

"An Alternative Approach to Allergies" by Theron G. Randolph. M.D. and Ralph W. Moss Ph.D. (Reference)

388

"The Fasting Cure" by Upton Sinclair. (Fun to read, reference)

"The Miracle Results of Fasting" by Dave Williams. (A little Christian book on fasting for health, and how to be closer to God)

A very good website for products, books and information is Gary Null's, Garynull.com

I found Livestrong.org to be a good source of information.

There are some movies about health on Netflix to be good and informative to watch.

Here are other sources of health information, which may be helpful to you.

"More Natural Cures Revealed" by Kevin Trudeau.

"How To Live Longer and Feel Better" by Linus Pauling. Also the Pauling institute online: http://lpi.oregonstate.edu

"Eating Well for Optimum Health" by Andrew Weil, M.D. (To read)

"The Glucose Revolution" by Jennie Brand-Miller: PhD. : Thomas M.S. Wolever, M.D., PhD: : Stephen Coagiuri, M.D. : Kaye Foster-Powell, M. Nut. & Diet. (To read)

"Enter the Zone" by Barry Sears, PhD, with Bill Lawren. (Emphasis is to use a proper ratio of proteins, carbohydrates and fats to be in the "zone" of mental and physical health).

More "King's Table Books"!

If you enjoyed this book, consider the other books in the "King's Table" series of books. The second book is "Protecting the King's Table" which has more about GMO foods and a complete listing of food additives to check on product labels. The third planned book is "Setting the King's Table" it is about how to cook healthy tasty foods including recipes.

To find these books search by title and author name. For instance, search on Amazon bookstore using "The King's Table" and Daniel W Osborne. Anyone who needs to speak to me can call 360-333-3709 or contact by email. Wretyduf@rocketmail.com, I am also on face book.

www.ingramcontent.com/pod-product-compliance
Lightning Source LLC
Chambersburg PA
CBHW072133290526
45794CB00004B/1301